MW01601217

SUZANNE BRACCI

HOPE for Struggling CATHOLICS

A Path to Spiritual & Personal Renewal

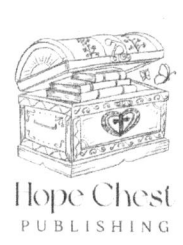

Hope Chest
PUBLISHING

First published by Hope Chest Publishing 2024

Copyright © 2024 by Suzanne Bracci

All rights reserved. No part of this publication may be reproduced, stored or transmitted in any form or by any means, electronic, mechanical, photocopying, recording, scanning, or otherwise without written permission from the publisher. It is illegal to copy this book, post it to a website, or distribute it by any other means without permission.

Suzanne Bracci asserts the moral right to be identified as the author of this work.

Suzanne Bracci has no responsibility for the persistence or accuracy of URLs for external or third-party Internet Websites referred to in this publication and does not guarantee that any content on such Websites is, or will remain, accurate or appropriate.

Designations used by companies to distinguish their products are often claimed as trademarks. All brand names and product names used in this book and on its cover are trade names, service marks, trademarks and registered trademarks of their respective owners. The publishers and the book are not associated with any product or vendor mentioned in this book. None of the companies referenced within the book have endorsed the book.

Scripture quotations marked KJV are from the King James Version of the Bible, which is in the public domain.

Scripture quotations marked NIV are taken from THE HOLY BIBLE, NEW INTERNATIONAL VERSION®, NIV® Copyright © 1973, 1978, 1984, 2011 by Biblica, Inc.® Used by permission. All rights reserved worldwide.

Scripture quotations marked NKJV are from the New King James Version®. Copyright © 1982 by Thomas Nelson. Used by permission. All rights reserved.

Scripture quotations marked NLT are taken from the Holy Bible, New Living Translation, copyright © 1996, 2004, 2015 by Tyndale House Foundation. Used by permission of Tyndale House Publishers, Inc., Carol Stream, Illinois 60188. All rights reserved.

First edition

ISBN: 979-8-9914152-0-0

Cover art by Amanda Bracci

This book was professionally typeset on Reedsy.
Find out more at reedsy.com

Contents

Dedication

I dedicate this book to my Mom, Barbara Donner Duran, for her tireless courage and commitment to her faith and her family.

Despite being widowed with five children under the age of ten and being eight months pregnant with her sixth child when her first husband, Charlie, passed away, she persevered and trusted God. She found her new husband, Richard, at a Catholic singles event. They had two more children, and our family quickly grew to ten people. Through it all, Mom was an energizer bunny, cooking meals every night of the week, and selflessly giving each of us her love, support, and attention. She devoted over 25 years of her life to volunteering as a religious education teacher while raising eight children.

While my Mom is still with us on this earth, she suffers from late-stage Alzheimer's disease and is not aware that I wrote this book. I know that if she knew, she would be my greatest supporter. I love you, Mom. May God bless you in your last years on this earth, and when the time comes, may Jesus welcome you into His heavenly glory. I love you now and forever, with endless gratitude.

Acknowledgments

A special thank you to my husband, Michael, for your love, patience, support, and trust that one day I would write "The End" on this book. To my children, Alexa, Justin, and Amanda, for your amazing love, support, and belief in me.

I am sincerely grateful to all my test readers: Linda Conlin, Fred Abbott, Teresa Casey, Lilia Bracci, Simona Kofanov, Nancy Galer, Patricia Gibson, Richard Duran, Theresa Smith, Susan Santandreu, Rev. Peter Drilling, Sr. Margaret Donner, Msgr. Paul Burkard, and Fr. Peter Santandreu. Thank you for devoting your time to reading my manuscript and offering wisdom, insight, edits, and suggestions.

Thank you to the countless people who shared their stories and supported me on this journey: Nancy, Patty, Nichelle, Simona, Theresa, Trish, Debbie, Paula, Elizabeth, Julie, Lynette, Sarah, Marie, Joe, Job, Pam, Jo Jo, Kathy, Gloria, Maria, Doreen, Brendan, Mary, Suzanne, Jane, Lori, and my Christ Renews His Parish Sisters-in-Christ.

A heartfelt thank you to my talented daughter, Amanda Bracci, for her beautiful hand-painted artwork and design of the book cover.

Introduction

Perhaps you've been struggling in your Catholic faith more recently, or it's been years or decades since you've stepped into a church. You're not alone. It's not easy to be Catholic, and sometimes it can even feel quite impossible.

Many things that have happened within the Catholic Church have shaken people's faith and broken their trust. Church leaders and clergy who were believed to be appointed through the anointing of the Holy Spirit and acting in the name of Jesus Christ have grievously sinned against God, His Church, and His people. Massive changes are occurring within the framework of faith communities, including the closure of churches and the merging of parishes. The future is uncertain.

This is a courageous conversation about the challenges of being Catholic, misconceptions of the faith, and failings within the Church resulting from human frailty, but, more importantly, it is an exploration of why we have faith in the first place and how to move forward in faith, hope, and love for God, each other, and ourselves. I long for you to know that despite the sinful and fallen nature of people, we can still enjoy and benefit from the Catholic faith in a profound and beautiful way.

I desire to be real and not pretend that I'm a perfect Catholic. I have thoughts, questions, and concerns about my faith that I think a lot of other people (Catholics and non-Catholics) have too. This book is an exploration of those ideas that are in the hearts and minds of Catholics.

Sadly, they are either misunderstood or not asked publicly in a room full of Catholics for fear of being rejected, ostracized, or shunned. There are plenty of books and apologetics written by theologians and biblical scholars on these topics. I'm neither. I'm an ordinary cradle Catholic who desires to know and understand my faith better and help others on this journey too.

This book reflects my beliefs at this time. Considering that our beliefs constantly change and evolve based on the information we receive, our life experiences, our faith formation, and the wisdom we gain through these avenues, I may have a different perspective on these issues in the future. Please grant me grace as I open my heart to the world in the hope that others may heal from past hurts and grow in their love for God and embrace (or at least appreciate) the Catholic faith.

I pray that through this book, *HOPE For Struggling CATHOLICS*, you will be uplifted and inspired to know how much God loves you. No matter what has happened in your life or how distant from your faith you might be, nothing can ever separate you from the love of Christ. Every moment of every day is a new opportunity to take one step closer to the love of God. I pray for you that God will give you strength for the journey and a life of abundant peace and joy.

May the love and peace of Christ be with you,

Suzanne

1

A "Good Catholic"

"And it is my prayer that your love may abound more and more, with knowledge and all discernment, so that you may approve what is excellent, and so be pure and blameless for the day of Christ" (Phil 1:9-10 NIV).

What Is a "Good Catholic?"

I've struggled my whole life to feel like a "good enough" Catholic. I grew up in a good Catholic home with strong morals and values and supportive parents. We went to church every Sunday and attended all the holy day masses. My siblings and I made all our sacraments, attended Catholic elementary school, attended Confession regularly, and prayed the rosary on every vacation road trip. I had the wonderful privilege of being a religious education teacher or volunteering in some capacity for the Church since my late teens. How could I, having done all this, still feel like a "not-good-enough" Catholic?

I could blame other people for this misfortune. I could say it's because a priest yelled at me in the confessional at eight years old. I could use the excuse that I had mean nuns who never seemed pleased with our class behavior. I could blame adults who expected me to be a perfectly obedient, rule-following Catholic young lady. Even when I didn't say the Hail Mary loud enough, I was scorned.

You see, I was born in the late 1960s, just a few years after the Second Vatican Council convened. This council, often referred to as Vatican II, marked a pivotal time in the history of the Church when the process of renewal and reform was initiated. Even though this period of reform emphasizing a more personal relationship with God had begun, the emphasis on strict adherence to rules, rituals, and moral codes remained the primary focus of Catholic teaching in many churches, religious education programs, and homes across the globe. Almost 60 years later, the effects of pre-Vatican II theology and education are still lingering in the minds, hearts, and practices of some Catholics. It's not anyone's fault; rather, it's just the way some things evolve... very slowly. I wish I had known growing up how much God loved me, just as I was, and that He saw my efforts, and they made Him happy.

I grew up feeling like it was nearly impossible to be a good Catholic. I couldn't be obedient enough, knowledgeable enough, or proactive enough to please many of the adult Catholic influences in my life. It just never felt like enough. I went through life thinking, "If I feel this way, do others feel this way too?" Over the years, and significantly more recently, I began to talk with other adult "cradle Catholics," those who are still attending Sunday Mass and those who are not practicing. I realized that we have many of the same things in common; this feeling of never quite making the mark, questioning and not having a clear understanding of some of the teachings, and experiencing Catholic guilt.

Catholic Guilt

Catholic guilt is real and pervasive. "Go to church every Sunday, attend all holy day masses, go to confession for the forgiveness of our sins, follow the 10 Commandments, pray the rosary, say grace before meals, and the list goes on." Yes, as Catholics, we are expected to do a lot. And when we don't do it, the guilt can set in. I've experienced multiple situations that compiled more feelings of guilt, resulting in not feeling "good enough" rather than feeling great about my faith. I'd like to tell you a few of those stories.

When I was in third grade, and attending Catholic elementary school, our whole class went to church for the Sacrament of Confession. It was shortly after I made my first Reconciliation, so I was a "newbie" to this. It was my least favorite part of my faith thus far, and it made me very anxious to tell the priest all of (what I viewed as) my "bad" qualities.

Before I went into the confessional, I recited the Act of Contrition over and over so that I would have it memorized and be able to recite it at the end of my time with the priest. Everything was going fine until after I confessed my sins. I couldn't think of anything else to tell him, so I was silent. The priest was silent. I was silent. The priest was silent. This silence went on for minutes. It seemed like 15 minutes, and I'm sure it wasn't that long, but it was definitely a very long period of silence. I thought to myself, "Did he leave the confessional?"

I began to get more and more anxious and didn't know if I should say anything. I thought to myself, isn't he supposed to talk next? I was timid and insecure. I just wanted to do it right. The next thing I knew, the priest sternly asked me if I was done telling him my sins. When I said "yes," he yelled at me telling me I had done it wrong and said I was supposed to tell him when I was done confessing my sins. He proceeded to ask where I learned how to go to Confession and told me that I didn't know the right way to do it. He said he would be talking to my teacher. I could tell that he was very agitated and frustrated with me.

Tears welled up in my eyes, and I had a huge lump in my throat, but I needed to hold it together. I needed to walk back to the pew past all of my classmates still in line. I mustered up the courage and held back the tears. As I walked past the line of classmates, one male classmate said, "You were in there forever! What did you do, Sue, knife a man?" I could not hold it together. It was the worst Catholic school memory I had.

Years later, when I was in the confessional and after sharing my sins and remorse, the priest told me that I shouldn't feel so bad about my sins and to "lighten up." "Wait a minute," I thought to myself. "What? Lighten up? Aren't I supposed to be remorseful for my sins?" Did the priest just ridicule me? That's what it seemed anyway, or maybe I just had a little post-traumatic stress from my previous confessional experience. Perhaps I wasn't forgiving myself. Maybe he wanted me to believe that Jesus had forgiven me. Whatever the reason he said that a better approach could have been taken. There is so much to contemplate. The message we receive is often influenced not only by a person's words but also by the tone of voice in their communication. For good or bad, it all affects our perception of a situation. I wish I had known then that people, even clergy, are imperfect, and that I shouldn't take things so seriously.

Unfortunately, millions of Catholics have suffered from guilt, mostly at their own expense. God wants us to be remorseful but not languish in long-term guilt and shame. Guilt is often the result of a misguided perception about what we think we need to do or should be. Guilt frequently stems from remorse for not living up to a certain standard or expectation, or disappointing someone else.[1] We feel guilt when we aren't sure that we are forgiven, and this could stem from us not believing that God truly has the power and grace to forgive us, or we just don't forgive ourselves. Either way, suffering from long-term guilt is not the plan that God has for us.

On the other hand, remorse resulting from short-term guilt or a "guilty conscience" can be very helpful. This conviction of the heart can be a sign that we need to look within. Perhaps God is calling us to some type of personal conversion or change. According to a Catholic Digest article "Grappling with guilt: The gift of God's GPS,"[2] guilt can be healthy or unhealthy. Healthy guilt is an invitation to look within, evaluate our lives, and make the necessary changes to heal physically, mentally, emotionally, or spiritually. The article describes healthy guilt as a blessing and sign that we need to course-correct and turn back to God so that we can fully experience His presence, peace, and joy. Unhealthy guilt reveals the need for healing on a deeper level.

Whether we suffer from short-term (healthy) or long-term (unhealthy) guilt, God calls us to take initiative. It's important to evaluate our guilt to determine if we need to make a change toward holiness or seek restoration through healing. We cannot wait passively and hope that those feelings will resolve themselves. God is on our side. He's waiting for us to turn to Him today so that we can experience true freedom and peace.

PRAYER: "Lord Jesus, help us to see the vastness of your love and mercy. Help us to recognize the difference between the guilt and shame that harms us and the conviction of the heart that guides us toward conversion and unity with you."

VERSE: "Godly sorrow brings repentance that leads to salvation and leaves no regret, but worldly sorrow brings death" (2 Cor 7:10).

Is Being a "Good Catholic" Important?

Over the years, as I strive to grow in knowledge and understanding of my faith, I often wonder, "What does it take to be a 'good Catholic,' and is this even important and achievable?" "Should I focus so much on 'doing things right,' as I learned growing up, or is there more to this faith journey?"

I had this nagging feeling that going through the motions just to "check the box" was meaningless without a heartfelt desire to know, love, and serve God. I knew there had to be a connection to the heart—a genuine longing to know Jesus and to pray, not just say, my prayers.

From a very young age, I've tried to do everything right. I said my prayers every night, went to church every Sunday with my family, sang in the church choir in elementary school, attended religious education classes, went to a Catholic elementary school, observed holy days, and received all my sacraments. I felt the presence of God many times throughout my childhood, and these practices developed a routine and commitment to my faith. However, there seemed to be more of a focus on doing things right and following the rules rather than fostering a personal friendship with God.

At one point, though, I thought I might have received a calling to become a nun. I was a young girl and remember enjoying playtime in the basement, where I could create magical worlds and become anything I wanted to be. I recall pretending to be a nun, placing a cloth on my head to represent a veil, holding my hands in prayer, and quietly pacing back and forth, pretending to be (and then finding myself) deep in prayer. It was a beautiful, magical time. Looking back, I feel like I experienced the presence of Jesus and such peace and calm when I transported myself in mind and spirit to serve God and His Church as a religious sister. What a beautiful moment in my life and early faith that was. I wasn't "checking" something off the box to be a "good Catholic."

I was having a personal encounter with God, and it was beautiful.

I continued my devout practice of the faith by serving as a religious education teacher in my 20s, and in my 30s, on the Liturgy of the Word committee and as a Vacation Bible School teacher. In my 40s, I attended Mission and became a Confirmation teacher. In my 50s, I attended and led a Christ Renews His Parish "Welcome" Retreat. I can't take all the credit for being so involved, though. I grew up in a home where we diligently practiced the faith and were expected to volunteer and serve our community. I had a strong foundation instilled in me to be a devout and "obedient" Catholic from an early age. While it wasn't easy and I often felt like I wasn't doing enough, I am very grateful to my mom and stepdad for their diligent efforts to raise my siblings and me to be good people with a solid moral Catholic Christian foundation. I learned the importance of volunteer work and serving our community, which helped me become caring, responsible, and committed to my faith.

So, what does it take to be a "good Catholic?" Is this even something important to strive for? Is it achievable? Shouldn't we love God and each other first and not worry so much about doing things "right?" We will explore those very questions and many more in this book

I am coming to realize that the reason we participate in any Christian faith denomination rests in a heartfelt desire to know, love, and serve God, becoming more and more like Him each day. It involves the heart as much as, if not more than, the mind. I don't think being a "good Catholic" means we have to be perfect in the human sense of being without flaws or understanding everything completely. I believe it involves earnestly striving to understand the doctrines and beliefs of the Church and not being afraid to question the things we don't yet understand. It involves continual change and growth. In fact, one of the great Christian authors of the 19th century, John Henry Newman, wrote in 1845: "In a higher world it is otherwise, but here below to live is to change and to be perfect is to have changed often."[3]

Growing close to God is a lifelong process. So too, is making Jesus Christ the center of our lives through practicing one's faith. No one should ever feel unworthy to practice their faith, as we are all sinners on this journey of growing, learning, and understanding our faith (and the purpose of it) more and more each day.

PRAYER: "Jesus, as we learn, grow, and even question our faith, please help us to have a heart that seeks your wisdom and truth. Please help us to practice our faith in a way that is pleasing to you. Amen."

VERSE: "If any of you lacks wisdom, you should ask God, who gives generously to all without finding fault, and it will be given to you" (James 1:5).

Human Perfection Isn't Realistic

"As for God, his way is perfect: The Lord's word is flawless; he shields all who take refuge in him" (Ps 18:30).

As I contemplate my Catholic faith, the questions that go through my mind are things like: "Is the Catholic Church looking for 100% compliance? Are we 'bad' Catholics if we question some of the Church's doctrines or beliefs? Can we still be 'good' Catholics if we don't believe in everything the Church teaches?"

Regarding 100% compliance, people are not robots to be programmed what to think and what to believe. I think it's quite impossible for people, with different life experiences, upbringings, and influences to understand things equally and believe the same exact thing. Yet informational sources such as Catholicscomehome.com state, "If we don't believe in all of it, if we appoint ourselves Pope and throw out a doctrine here or a doctrine there, then our faith is no longer Catholic."[4] I had an agnostic say to me, one time, "If Catholics do not believe 100% in everything the Church teaches, they're not Catholic then." Wow. That's a lot to ponder.

If one says that, then one is looking for perfection, and that's unachievable. Only God is perfect. How can we be realistic with ourselves and others? How can everyone be treated with love and acceptance, with the realization that everyone is at varying levels of belief and faith?

That's an essential question that must be thought about. Love, acceptance, and having realistic expectations for one another as God's children is critical. Supporting, encouraging, and educating each other with gentleness and humility, along the way, is necessary. It can't be "I'm right, and you're wrong." It can't be, "I know everything about Catholicism, and here's what you need to know." It can't be rudeness, put-downs, or pride, as I and others have experienced with some Catholics we've encountered. It can't be any of that, or people will turn away from the Church, feeling unworthy and unwelcome. The reality is that we're all unworthy, but with God's grace, mercy, and forgiveness, we can all feel welcome to come to the table of the Lord and be strengthened by His redeeming love.

So, how does one reach the point of feeling worthy to be Catholic? Is this even important to be thinking about? I've met devout practicing Catholics who are so bewildered at this time. They are confused about what to believe and who to trust. They question their Catholic faith. Some cling to what they know and what they love about the Church. They love the Mass, they love the sacraments, and they love receiving Holy Communion. I think this is beautiful. We need to rejoice and be glad that not everyone is leaving the Church despite the tragedies that have occurred. Catholics need to regain hope and trust in the Church.

The Church needs to be welcoming and meet people where they're at. There will be many different points of view on the journey, and they're all okay. Let me say that again... they're all okay.

We are a community of believers standing together, not standing alone one by one. Imagine us linking arms, one person at a time, adding another and another, until our chain of unity grows so big that it encompasses our family, our community, our state, and eventually the whole globe. We have to start somewhere. And it begins with each and every one of us.

PRAYER: "Lord, help us to have realistic expectations for ourselves and others. Help us to be gentle and humble of heart, loving others and working together to build your Church here on earth as we grow in holiness and love for you. Amen."

VERSE: "Do nothing out of selfish ambition or vain conceit. Rather, in humility value others above yourselves, not looking to your own interests but each of you to the interests of the others" (Phil 2:3-4).

Strive for Progress, Not Perfection

"Be diligent in these matters; give yourself wholly to them, so that everyone may see your progress" (1 Tim 4:15).

Perfectionism is a myth that destroys peace and hope. When we strive for perfection, we attempt to achieve something that is ultimately impossible. It is a dangerous and painful place to live. I would claim myself to be a recovering perfectionist, someone who was always striving and working towards perfection. It's a trap for frustration, disappointment, and discontentment.

Neither people nor the Catholic Church can ever be perfect. In fact, no denomination, business, organization, or school is, or can ever be, perfect. Sin and corruption are evident in all these places because they are all led by human beings with faults, shortcomings, and free will. We can't look at any of them with the eyes of perfection, because it's simply not possible. As far as being a Catholic Christian goes, if perfect understanding and 100% compliance with all of the doctrines and teachings are expected, we will isolate and ostracize everyone who does not fit the mold. It saddens me. It concerns me. I don't think that's God's heart, or the goal of Catholicism or Christianity at all, yet there are remnants of this mentality still present in the Catholic Church.

Since there is "No condemnation for those who are in Christ Jesus" (Romans 8:1), how did we somehow think we had to be perfect and feel guilty when we're not? This is not what God teaches us. We need to rise above the Catholic guilt and let it affect us no more. I'm not saying we shouldn't strive to be excellent human beings. I believe it's important to live a virtuous life of integrity and love for God while following biblical teachings. I'm not saying we shouldn't look within and strive to make changes to continually better ourselves, because that is an important thing to do, but striving for perfection in our human strength is an impossible task. "Jesus looked at them and said, 'With man this is impossible, but with God all things are possible'" (Matt 19:26). We will never be perfect. Only God is perfect.

Maybe faith isn't about being a "good enough" Catholic at all. Although I learned, while growing up, that following the rules and doctrine to perfection was the goal of the Catholic Christian life, I now realize this is a misunderstanding. Does this mean we go AWOL, denying our faith and the beauty, richness, and truth found in the Catholic Church and its teachings? No. Does it mean we pick the pieces we want to believe and disregard the rest? No, not necessarily. What I am suggesting is that we keep learning and growing in our faith every day.

We must invest some time and energy into our faith to expand our understanding and to continue to grow spiritually in wisdom and grace. There are many ways of understanding and explaining each of our beliefs, and we won't understand things the same or agree with everyone. It's impossible. Find a reputable Catholic scholar whose viewpoints are similar to yours and who explains things in a way that makes sense to you. I have learned not to let the confusion, disbelief, or frustration be in the driver's seat but rather to be curious, a continual learner, and have an open mind to pursue the truth.

Christian perfection is not about achieving human perfection or following rules and doctrine to an exact science, but rather, it is about seeking God's perfect and pleasing will. "Be perfect, therefore, as your heavenly Father is perfect" (Matt 5:48). As I get older (and hopefully wiser) I am coming to realize that faith is about total reliance on God and a "completeness" in Him alone. It is about knowing, loving, and serving God with all my heart, soul, mind, and strength. It is a call to repentance and conformity, one step at a time, day by day, to the will of God. My religious practices are a vehicle for getting me there.

PRAYER: "God, you are the center of our lives. Help us to focus on you first in all that we do. Help us to put religion in the right context so that we are seeking you and your will above all other things. Amen."

VERSE: "But seek first his kingdom and his righteousness, and all these things will be given to you as well" (Matt 6:33).

2

A Broken Church & Heart

"Therefore, among God's churches, we boast about your perseverance and faith in all the persecutions and trials you are enduring" (2 Thess 1:4).

Shattered Trust

The clergy abuse scandal and mishandling of these cases by Church authorities made me re-evaluate everything I believed and trusted about my faith. It made me question who I could trust and second-guess just about everything I had learned. I was devastated and deeply saddened, especially for those most vulnerable who were affected. For a time, I was even embarrassed to identify myself as Catholic in public, fearing it might turn other Christians away. I felt bewildered and uncertain about my commitment to the Catholic faith. Our whole community of believers was distraught, especially when our very own pastor was found guilty of abuses himself. Even worse, one of my family members was a victim of grooming by this priest, though, thankfully, he was able to escape each time.

The Catholic Church is in crisis around the United States and the world due to the abuse scandal and several other challenges. Many dioceses are facing a significant priest shortage, declining Mass attendance, and aging congregations. In my diocese, it was announced that approximately one-third of parishes would be closing their church buildings and merging with other parishes.[5] At the time of this writing, thirty-five Catholic dioceses and religious organizations across the United States have sought Chapter 11 bankruptcy protection.[6] In October of 2023, my diocese reported that it would have to pay 100 million dollars in reparations to the victims of the clergy abuse.[7] Many dioceses throughout the United States are facing the same problem. This is a lot to take in. I don't blame parishioners for being angry about this. On one hand, why should faithful parishioners pay for the sins of the priests? On the other hand, as members of a community that supports and helps one another, isn't it important to come together in love, responsibility, and commitment to make things right and move past this painful time in the life of our Church?

Douglas J. Lucia, the Syracuse Bishop, was quoted in an article saying, "As a Catholic family, it is our moral obligation to provide reparation and share a role in bringing healing and reconciliation to the survivors."[8] This is a hard pill to swallow for Catholics who have been faithfully contributing to their church and feel betrayed. We are humans with feelings, opinions, frustrations, anger, and a plethora of other emotions. How do we move past those feelings to a place of trust and love for our Church once again? How do we get to a place where we are okay with paying for the sins of the priests? Is this something we ought to even think about doing?

When a business or organization does something unethical, people often send a clear message that they don't support those actions by boycotting that business or organization. I've met people who are taking that stand with the Catholic Church. I understand their stance. It was embarrassing for a while to associate with the Catholic Church, fearing that by supporting the Church and remaining a contributing member, I would send the message that I supported what had happened. It's uncomfortable to be in this position. It is disheartening and disappointing. How do we repair the wounds, compensate the survivors, learn from this, and move on stronger than before?

This is not easy, and it will take the Church leadership's dedicated effort to take full responsibility for the heinous crimes committed. This is a difficult time in the history of the Church, and it is indeed a sad and disturbing time. My heart breaks for all people directly and indirectly impacted.

This isn't really something new, though. The Church has experienced injustices at the hands of its leaders for centuries and, in many ways, has been "broken" for over 2,000 years. Looking back, several controversial practices within the Catholic Church have defiled its reputation and eroded believers' confidence. Some of these practices included selling reduced punishment for sins (indulgences), favoring relatives to religious positions regardless of merit (nepotism), buying or selling spiritual offices, sacraments, or church roles (simony), and holding multiple Church offices often for power or income (pluralism) which led to neglect of pastoral responsibilities (absenteeism).[9] The Church became exposed, and its leaders had to make things right. These injustices cannot and should not be hidden, pushed under a rug, or made light of. They create division and a lack of trust and confidence. The Church needs to take accountability and responsibility and make things right. We are at another critical time when the Church must examine its motives, reform efforts, and rebuild trust.

PRAYER: "Lord Jesus, life can be confusing and cruel. We live in a fallen

*world where sin and corruption exist all around us, but we know that you
have the final word. Your word is light and truth in this dark world, and we
put our trust in you. Show us the way forward. Amen."*

*VERSE: "Behold, God is my salvation; I will trust, and will not be afraid; for
the Lord God is my strength and my song, and he has become my salvation"
(Isa 12:2).*

People Are Imperfect, but God Isn't

*"For the foolishness of God is wiser than human wisdom, and the weakness of
God is stronger than human strength" (1 Cor 1:25 NIV).*

The clergy abuse scandal was a pivotal point in my faith journey where
I realized that no one is perfect or all-knowing except God. Priests,
bishops, cardinals, deacons, and all other religious leaders are not
immune to failings and sin. I feel foolish and naive for having believed
that clergy and religious leaders were like God on earth, as I was taught.

While clergy have the same human frailties as the laity, I believe most
have divine graces given to them by God to lead with God's purposes
as their primary intent. I believe they have a genuine calling and pure
desire to love and serve God and His people. In fact, studies show
that the overwhelming majority (96%) of priests were not a part of
the clergy abuse scandal.[10] Make no mistake, 4% is way too many,
and this has been a tragedy in the Church. It will take a miracle and
the grace of God to repair the suffering of those impacted and their
families, turning the hatred and pain into forgiveness and healing.
Of the 4% involved in the scandal, I believe many did not choose
the priesthood for the right reasons. I know of one such priest who
was told that he had two choices: either join the priesthood or go to

jail. Not the best way to choose to enter the priesthood, is it. Today, there are stricter seminary entrance requirements. Applicants undergo screening processes, including written psychological tests and personal interviews, that help ensure that the man is psychologically and mentally ready to enter the seminary. They don't just "get in," and it is a rigorous process to be accepted into theological studies programs and prepare for the priesthood. This is a step in the right direction.

How do we move forward with honor for religious leaders and clergy without expecting them to be perfect like God? The answer, I believe, is knowing the difference between human religious leaders, who are earthen vessels, and Jesus Christ. "For the law appoints as high priests men in all their weakness; but the oath, which came after the law, appointed the Son, who has been made perfect forever" (Heb 7:28).

God gave His son, Jesus Christ, as a ransom for all to show us the way, the truth, and the life. Jesus is our one true North Star, our Savior, and the reason for everything in existence. We can stay grounded in the truth by studying holy Scripture, following His teachings, and engaging in prayer and worship. Remember that God is the only one we need to please. We should never seek to please people unless we feel the prompting of the Holy Spirit to do so. Even in that case, pleasing God always comes before anything else. This is confirmed in Colossians 3:23, where it reads: "Whatever you do, work at it with all your heart, as working for the Lord, not for human masters."

Our faithful priests are suffering from the sins of their brothers in Christ. They need our love, compassion, support, and prayers. Their calling and job is not an easy one. There are fewer and fewer priests now who have more and more responsibilities added to their already busy ministry schedule. One of the most beautiful ministries to support our priests is the Seven Sisters Apostolate. It has been a blessing to be a part of this ministry and a joy and honor to pray for my parish's pastor. By spending one hour in prayer each week over the last year, my faith and closeness with God have increased exponentially. I have experienced the true peace of Christ sitting in my church, often all alone, in front of the Tabernacle or Eucharist. What a beautiful holy experience. I encourage other parishes around the world to adopt this ministry. All it takes is the willing hearts of seven women in the parish to commit to praying for the pastor, one person each day of the week for one hour for one year. To learn more about this ministry, go to https://sevensistersapostolate.org/.[11]

PRAYER: *"Lord, in our sadness and distress, help us remember that your strength is made perfect in our weakness. Nothing is too difficult for you. Help us trust in you to heal our wounds and the wounds of your people."*

VERSE: *"Nevertheless, I will bring health and healing to it; I will heal my people and will let them enjoy abundant peace and security" (Jer 33:6).*

The Need for Continual Reform

"Strengthen what remains and is about to die" (Rev 3:2).

We must take a look at our practices and beliefs, and continually evaluate them. This practice is called "Ecclesia semper reformanda," a Latin phrase commonly associated with the Catholic Church, meaning "the Church must always be reformed."[12] In a catholicculture.org article, Bishop R. Walter Nickless states,

> The Church is always in need of renewal because it is made up of us, imperfect human beings. This is the deepest reason: as individuals and as a Church, we are always called to grow, change, deepen, repent, convert, improve, and learn from our

successes and failures in the pursuit of holiness and fidelity to Jesus Christ and the mission He has given us. Moreover, we need to do this in the midst of an ever changing world, culture and society.[13]

The Church is constantly evolving and in need of improvement. Ongoing reform and renewal are necessary to adapt to changing times and circumstances. The tough question is, "How can we do this while remaining true to our core beliefs and teachings?" I believe Pope Francis is striving to do this. In his book, *A Gift of Joy and Hope*, he encourages readers to foster inclusive attitudes and overcome division by recognizing the beauty in the world and every person. He calls us to change attitudes that exclude others.[14]

Looking back, thank God there were people like Martin Luther King Jr. and Rosa Parks who fought for equal rights and challenged laws and beliefs of the time. Even though segregation still existed, people challenged those mainstream beliefs and practices, and now we have more equality. Is this a time for more equality again? Should we be welcoming the LGBTQ+ community with open arms? They are equally God's children. I don't know all the answers; I'm just asking the question. We must consider what is noble, right, and praiseworthy in God's eyes (Phil 4:8).

Even within the Catholic Church, there is a vast difference in opinions and beliefs. I am frustrated as I imagine many are over the controversy within the Church and among its leaders. How are we supposed to know what to think, and who to believe or trust when there is so much division within the Church? Wouldn't God want us to find common ground? Simply listening to various Catholic speakers also presents one with a smorgasbord of viewpoints that often even oppose each other. This presents a real dilemma for Catholics who want to do what is right in the eyes of God and understand Catholic Church teaching.

As we move forward, desiring a more unified Church grounded in the love and example of Christ and His Church, may we remember the vital role we each play in building the Church within our hearts, minds, families, and communities. May we remember to trust in the Lord, and not rely on our own understanding (Prov 3:5) as we submit to His will.

PRAYER: "Lord God, help us realize that only you are perfect and that we cannot expect perfection from anything led by human beings. Direct our paths to be an instrument of positive change and reform within our sphere of influence and help us to be patient as we accept the things we cannot change. Guide our Church to reform and change according to your will. Amen."

VERSE: "For my thoughts are not your thoughts, neither are your ways my ways," declares the Lord. "As the heavens are higher than the earth, so are my ways higher than your ways and my thoughts than your thoughts" (Isa 55:8-9).

3

Healing and Moving Forward

"He heals the brokenhearted and binds up their wounds" (Ps 147:3).

First Steps

So where do we go from here, with so much dissension, mistrust, disillusionment, and confusion concerning the Catholic Church? How do we move on from the pain and betrayal? How do we recommit ourselves to a Church that is broken and run by humans who likely will make poor choices that grieve God over and over again?

I am immediately reminded of this Scripture passage: "Now faith is confidence in what we hope for and assurance about what we do not see" (Heb 11:1). Faith is the first essential ingredient.

If we are to move forward, some other essential things need to take place. First, we need to realize that people with imperfect hearts and minds run the Catholic Church and all institutions. Second, we must put our trust in God, our creator, not man. Third, we need to pray for those in leadership roles in the Church and not condemn all for the sins of some. Fourth, we need to acknowledge the role of the Holy Spirit as our source of hope and path to conversion. Despite the sinfulness, errors, and mistakes that the human part of our Church may make, we live under the protection and guidance of the Holy Spirit, who, through grace, gives us hope for a better future and, somehow, shows us a path to conversion, and a more perfect way to be His people, His Church on earth.

To move forward, we must also recognize the lies of the enemy who wants to keep us as far as possible from our faith and love for God. The enemy, Satan, the prince of darkness and source of all evil, would love to keep us stuck in anger and separation from our faith and the Church forever. He will do what he can to keep us stuck there. We need to be aware of and recognize the lies of Satan, including situations and emotions he uses to separate us from God's love. The great news is that "the things which are impossible with men are possible with God" (Luke 18:27). When we put God in the driver's seat and allow the Holy Spirit to guide us, HOPE and healing are always within reach.

PRAYER: "God, we put our faith and trust in you alone. Open our eyes to see how we can move forward in hope and healing."

VERSE: "Let the morning bring me word of your unfailing love, for I have put my trust in you. Show me the way I should go, for to you I entrust my life" (Ps 143:8).

Three Lies that Prevent Healing

When we allow certain emotions, such as anger, pride, and fear, to camp out in our hearts and minds, there is a schism between us and God's healing power. Consequently, the grace of hope and healing is difficult to achieve. We all want to move forward and heal from past hurts. No one wants to stay stuck in anger and resentment. Pride and fear also lead us astray, taking us further from the love, peace, and hope in Christ that we desire.

Anger

Anger is a normal emotion. We all feel and experience it when we are betrayed, mistreated, ignored, or lied to. It is normal, healthy, and natural for anger to arise during situations such as these. Let me be clear. We have a right to be angry about the sins of clergy and religious leaders who we trusted. It is normal to be angry if we are mistreated or ostracized from our church family. Anger isn't all bad, and there are benefits to anger. Anger can protect us from danger and alert us when we need to take action or seek justice or resolution to a problem. From a mental health and social/emotional perspective, however, anger is not an emotion that we ought to allow to reside in our minds and hearts for an extended period of time. Why not? Here are 10 reasons:

1. Anger steals our peace and joy
2. Anger can turn to resentment and fuel strife in relationships
3. Anger can make us seek revenge
4. Anger can make us say things that we later regret
5. Anger impacts our thoughts which impacts our emotions
6. Anger can lead to hopelessness
7. Anger negatively impacts our mental health and can lead to anxiety
8. Anger impacts both our home and work life
9. Anger affects our quality of life and enjoyment of the present moment
10. Anger is a form of pride

We need to work through our anger so that it does not become resentment, bitterness or strife. These are not fruits of the Holy Spirit but works of the flesh. It's important to avoid these and cling to God's Word and truth with all of our heart, mind, and soul. Through my time working in schools teaching social emotional skills and training adults in implementing character education programs, one of the things we taught is that "anger" is one step away from "danger" when you add the D. Why did we teach this? Because unresolved anger, with one little trigger, can lead to a behavior that is dangerous, hurtful, illegal, or deeply regrettable. God's word instructs us: "In your anger do not sin. Do not let the sun go down while you are still angry, and do not give the devil a foothold" (Eph 4:26-27).

Another problem with anger is when we hold onto it, it can lead to other emotions that turn from healthy to unhealthy. Anger has also been shown to increase levels of the stress hormone cortisol in the body which can be damaging in many ways. Stress increases heart rate, blood pressure, and immune response. These in turn increase the risk of anxiety, depression, heart attack, and stroke, among other conditions.[15]

Nelson Mandela once said "Resentment is like drinking poison and then hoping it will kill your enemies."[16] I believe that resentment is a form of pride that forms when we are hurt and we hold onto that hurt and anger toward the other person. It is a dark seed that is not in alignment with God's will for us. In fact, it's the opposite. God wishes us peace, joy, and fruitful loving relationships.

Regarding anger and resentment, of course, we can't just wish those emotions away. Wouldn't that be nice? By processing and discussing our feelings with loved ones, especially Godly Christians, we can put them into perspective in a healthier, more forward-moving manner. Seek Godly counsel from friends. Be cautious of those who will be "problem-focused," feeding our anger and resentment. Seek professional help from a counselor or life coach for struggles that are difficult to let go of, preventing resolution and peace. I recommend finding someone with a Christian, solution-focused, and biblical approach.

The more we stay stuck in the past, in disappointment and anger, the longer it will take to move on. What I'm suggesting is to be future-oriented, thinking more about solutions than past problems. Cling to optimism and a hopeful perspective that God knows everything we're going through and will work it out for good. God's Word promises the following things...

- "And we know that in all things God works for the good of those who love him, who have been called according to his purpose" (Rom 8:28).
- "I will instruct you and teach you in the way you should go; I will counsel you with my loving eye on you" (Ps 32:8).

I'd like to tell you a story of when anger and resentment got the best of me. I was a middle school counselor at the time, diligently working late to answer all the emails and return parent phone calls. It was around 5:20 PM, and I was finishing up for the day when I started to hear loud noises in the school. All the principals, counselors, and administrative assistants had gone home for the day and I was the last person in the office.

I started to hear loud noises in the building, like desks being overturned and shouting in the hallways. I waited for a time to see if the noises stopped and decided to peek into the hallway. To my shock, a man was standing a mere 8 feet away from me pointing what looked like a rifle at me in a "shoot to kill" position. He did not lower the gun and remained silent as he held that gun at me. I frantically ran into my office, shut the door, and hid under the desk. All that went through my mind was "Could this be my last day on this earth?"

As I crouched there in fright, I decided to call both secretaries, but neither one knew of a drill. At that moment, gunshots reamed out, one after another, as the shouting, running, and violent noises in the halls intensified. I immediately called 911 to get help. As I waited on the call for the 911 intake person to come back, I shivered in fear as I thought, "Might I die at the hands of this shooter?" and "Will I see my husband and children again?"

As the 911 operator came back on the phone, I could not believe what I heard her say…"Ma'am, I'm really sorry, but the local police are doing an active shooter drill in the school building. You will be fine and can go home." "I will be fine? What, go home?" I thought with exasperation and anger. The sound of gunshots continued to pierce my ears as the supposed drill continued for several minutes.

It was the scariest day of my life and, what's worse, I called the school principal on my car ride home to tell him what happened and he said he had no knowledge of a drill but it was possible that a notification could be within his 300 unchecked emails. I was livid. I can't tell you all that happened after that because it would take up half this book, but I can tell you that I was beside myself in anger toward the people who neglected to inform me about the active shooter drill.

Negative thoughts pervaded my mind for weeks and even months as I tried to heal and move forward from this traumatic event. I was reminded of it every time I passed that section of the hallway to enter my office. I was suffering from post-traumatic stress and knew it could have been prevented if people had been more responsible in notifying me of this drill.

The resentment and bitterness were eating away at me. Self-pity had settled into my heart, and I learned firsthand the truth about what a devouring spirit self-pity is. I knew I had to release this, turn to God, and change my negative thoughts to be more positive and productive. I cared very much about my students and doing my job to the best of my ability. To do that I needed to confront and then forgive the people responsible and move on.

Thank goodness through faith, prayer, and the repetition of positive affirmations, along with a few therapy sessions, I was able to move forward and let it go. Living in the past did not serve me well, and I doubt it will ever serve you well either.

In the same way, as difficult as it is, we need to find a way to move past any anger, bitterness, and resentment we feel toward the Church or its people. Holding onto our anger and self-pity will only make things worse, but resolving these feelings will bring peace to our minds and hearts and better health to our bodies.

PRAYER: "Lord, guide us to find a way to resolve feelings of anger, bitterness, and strife. You want us to live a life of peace and joy, and we know this is possible with your help."

VERSE: "My dear brothers and sisters, take note of this: Everyone should be quick to listen, slow to speak and slow to become angry, because human anger does not produce the righteousness that God desires" (Jam 1:19-20).

Pride

God's word instructs us that "Pride brings a person low, but the lowly in spirit gain honor" (Prov 19:23). The Oxford English Dictionary (OED) defines pride as "an excessively high opinion of one's own worth or importance which gives rise to a feeling or attitude of superiority over others; inordinate self-esteem."[17] Pride can lead to arrogance, and result in treating others as if they are "less important" than ourselves. It is a dangerous place to be and can adversely affect our relationships with others, and especially our relationship with God, giving rise to the belief that we are self-sufficient and not in need of a Savior in Jesus Christ.

Instead of behaving in a way that allows pride to be in the driver's seat, I believe we must deny our ego satisfaction and live each day exemplifying humility in our thoughts, words, and actions. "When pride comes, then comes disgrace, but with humility comes wisdom" (Prov 11:2).

To be humble does not mean we sit back and allow other people to walk all over us. Humility does not mean we don't stand up for what we believe in. Humility is recognizing that all people are equal in importance and that one is no better than anyone else. It's important not to look down on anyone else who has sinned, such as Church clergy and leaders (as difficult as that is), because we, too, are sinners. We all need God's mercy, love, forgiveness, and salvation. None of us are immune to sin. That's why we need Jesus as our Savior.

Pride separates us from unity with other people. Perhaps it is the one thing that has caused more people to leave the Church than anything else. We must be cautious of believing that somehow we are better or too good to be affiliated or associated with an organization that includes sinners in a leadership role. Sadly, when we do this, I think we are fooling ourselves. There are imperfect people prone to sin, making poor choices every day in every organization on planet Earth.

We need to accept our imperfect nature, unite, and help one another in this life journey to be the best we can be. The only way we can do this is to exercise humility. I recently read in Pope Francis' book "A Gift of Joy and Hope" that the only time we should be looking down on anyone else is to lend them a hand to help them back up.[18] What a beautiful expression of humility and a wonderful mantra to live up to. Scripture reminds us that "God opposes the proud, but gives grace to the humble" (James 4:6). Pride prevents us from seeking and experiencing healing. Humility opens the door for forgiveness and peace, hence restoring our faith and community of believers.

PRAYER: "Lord, search our hearts for areas of pride that limit us from being the person you have created us to be. Help us to grow in humility and love."

VERSE: "The end of a matter is better than its beginning, and patience is better than pride" (Eccl 7:8).

Fear

Fear is paralyzing. I've heard over and over that fear is the opposite of faith. I truly have come to believe that wholeheartedly. In my late 20s and early 30s, I was blessed to have the opportunity to attend a Bible study led by a beautiful Godly woman named Jody. During that time, my faith grew exponentially through studying Scripture, increasing my prayer life, and trusting God. Jody told us that the acronym F.E.A.R. stands for "False-Evidence-Appearing-Real." To me, that was very profound. It was during a time when I had many fears about being a working Mom and raising children. It was also an uncertain time when our family was traveling with my husband's job, which required us to pack our suitcases and move quite frequently. By clinging to God's promises in Scripture and remembering this FEAR acronym, I was able to keep my fears at bay and trust in God's loving provision and care.

What fears do you have that keep you stuck? What fears prevent you from healing and becoming your best self? What fears do you have about the Catholic Church or renewing your faith? Do you worry about not being good enough? God says, "Come as you are." He knows we are imperfect and says, "I love you just as you are." He invites us to "Come to me, all who labor and are heavy laden, and I will give you rest" (Matt 11:28).

The closer we are to God, the less we have to fear. It's the safest place we can be. God's Word verifies that "There is no fear in love. But perfect love drives out fear, because fear has to do with punishment. The one who fears is not made perfect in love" (1 John 4:18). Our God is loving and patient. "The LORD is gracious and full of compassion, Slow to anger and great in mercy" (Ps 145:8 NKJV).

There are many biblical references about the importance of not fearing and the wisdom to recognize fear for what it is. Know that it is not God's wish or will for us to live with fear, ever. In fact, it completely opposes God's will for how we live. When fear arises in our minds and emotions, it is essential to dismiss it as quickly as possible and recite Scripture such as "Fear not, for I am with you; be not dismayed, for I am your God; I will strengthen you, I will help you, I will uphold you with my righteous right hand" (Isa 41:10 NIV). How wonderful it is to know that "God has not given us a spirit of fear, but of power and of love and of a sound mind" (2 Tim 1:7 NKJV). Let us cling to this promise every day!

So, in review, three lies that hold us back from healing and being reunited with the truest love of God and our faith are anger, pride, and fear. May God uncover these areas for each of us, providing opportunities to experience His healing power and bringing humility, peace, and joy.

PRAYER: "Lord, uncover areas of fear that are harboring in our minds and hearts. Help us to embrace your healing love and cast out fear in accordance with your will so that we may heal and be free from this bondage."

VERSE: "I sought the Lord, and he answered me; he delivered me from all my fears. Those who look to him are radiant; their faces are never covered with shame" (Ps 34:4-5 NIV).

Distractions to Our Faith

Satan loves to keep us far from God, the Church, and our faith. He loves to plant dark seeds in our hearts that breed resentment, bitterness, despair, disillusionment, confusion, and disgust. His goal is to separate us as far as possible from our faith in God and the Church. Satan uses human frailty and sin as a tool to further separate us from the love of God and His Church. Satan is the king of lies and deception. For example, the sins and betrayal of clergy and those in religious leadership positions were the perfect vices for Satan to use to drive a wedge between God's people and their faith. Satan is very sly. He uses the human frailties of others as justification, in people's minds, to abandon and leave the faith.

Of course, in our human understanding, why would we stay affiliated with an organization or Church with corrupt leaders? It's very easy to justify in our minds that the right thing to do is to separate from such an organization. The problem with this thinking is that it is shortsighted and precisely the way Satan wants us to view the situation. He wants us to justify leaving. He delights in using the sins of religious people to drive away as many as he can from God's love, mercy, and saving power. These sins give him the perfect fuel to ignite doubt, discouragement, anger, bitterness, sadness, frustration, and hatred for the Church. Please be on guard for this, not in a fearful way, but in a mindful, observant way.

The sins of the clergy have become distractions to our faith. We have to separate the sins of people from the status of our faith. Our faith is in God alone, not in men. God's word reveals, "It is better to trust in the LORD than to put confidence in man" (Ps 118:8 KJV). Jeremiah 17:5 also warns us about putting our trust in humankind. This Scripture tells us, "Cursed is the one who trusts in man, who draws strength from mere flesh and whose heart turns away from the LORD" (NIV).

Separating from our religious community hurts us more than it hurts anyone else. We can say, "Well, they're not getting my money anymore," or "It serves the Church right for losing all these people because it betrayed us." We can say, "The Church secretary was so rude that it turned me off." We could come up with a hundred other reasons for leaving and being angry. They're all likely very valid reasons to feel hurt, disappointed, frustrated, and angry... on the surface. When we look beneath the surface though, we can usually see that the source of much of the pain and crisis in the Church is the result of human sin and frailty.

As I mentioned earlier, another distraction to our faith is feeling insecure or unworthy to practice our faith within a religious community. God's perfect love is understanding, and it casts out fear, insecurity, and doubt. God's perfect love is full of mercy and forgiveness. God's perfect love hopes for the best but expects the worst. He knows we are broken. He expects us to sin but also calls us to be our best selves each day. As international speaker and author Matthew Kelly says, "Be the best version of yourself." As far as being a Catholic Christian, I feel the best we can do is continue to grow in knowledge and understanding of our doctrine and beliefs and learn more about the ones we don't yet understand or truly 100% accept.

Many Catholics are upset by the closing and consolidation of parishes. In our diocese, this is called the "Road to Renewal." These changes can be very difficult to understand and accept. The pastors who were loved by many have now been moved to another parish. We are faced with re-organization and bankruptcy in many dioceses across the country. Some parishes that have been around for over 100 years are faced with their church building closing and merging with another "family of parishes." Parishioners are left wondering how they will find the same solace and faith-filled experience in a new church community and physical church space.

It can be truly disheartening, for sure. Let's not allow Satan to use this as another distraction to our faith. As difficult as it is, we must accept the changes and trust that God has a good plan for our Church. It will help to have faith, trusting that the Holy Spirit is guiding the process. I pray we can have hope in the future and pray for God to call good, righteous men of faith to enter the priesthood. Release expectations and control and give it to God. This will bring us peace and an assurance that the future is bright with hope and possibilities. No one knows what the future will bring. Only God does. As long as we stay close to His love and goodness and seek the guidance of the Holy Spirit, we will have the best chance of being on the right path in God's will.

What we choose to think about impacts every aspect of our lives. Focusing and perseverating on the sins of the clergy, the offenses done to us by church members and leaders, or the changes we don't like or agree with creates a wider gap in the love, peace, and joy Jesus promises us through our faith.

Reflection: What is one *distraction* to your faith that you want to let go of? How will you do that?

PRAYER: *"Lord Jesus, protect our minds and hearts. Keep us from the lies of the enemy and keep us close to the heart of Jesus. Help us recognize distractions to our faith and move beyond these obstacles so that we can experience the joy and contentment you provide. Amen."*

VERSE: *"Wait for the Lord; be strong and take heart and wait for the Lord"* (Ps 27:14).

Forgiveness

To experience healing and the fullness of joy in our relationships and faith, granting forgiveness is essential. God promises us, "If you forgive those who sin against you, your heavenly Father will forgive you" (Matt 6:14 NLT). God believes the best in us. God expects us to treat others as He is treating us, and that includes forgiveness. Forgiveness involves humility and a disposition of the heart that remembers we need forgiveness as much as everyone else. We all equally need forgiveness for our sins. He calls us to look within, discerning what personal conversion needs to occur before chastising another person for their sins. "You hypocrite, first take the plank out of your own eye, and then you will see clearly to remove the speck from your brother's eye" (Matt 7:5 NIV).

God gives us grace by forgiving our sins and expects us to extend that same grace to others by forgiving them. "Bear with each other and forgive one another if any of you has a grievance against someone. Forgive as the Lord forgave you" (Col 3:13). God knows this is not easy. Our human pain, wants, needs, and pride cloud the desire to want to forgive, but forgiveness brings peace.

Scripture paints a tall order in Matthew 5:44 to "Love your enemies and pray for those who persecute you." I believe this is one of the most significant challenges we are called to in all of Scripture...to love our enemies and pray for those who mistreat us. It seems counterintuitive and almost illogical. But God's ways always make sense in the end, even when they don't make sense in our human intellect.

When we remember that harboring anger and resentment is counterproductive to our health and well-being, it starts to make sense again. It's essential to be mindful of when we need to draw the line with anger and move to forgiveness. To hold onto it, how is that helpful? Does it bring resolution? Does it make us feel better? Maybe for a time. The

better question is, "How does it make us feel worse? How does it keep us stuck in a state of disillusionment, disgust, depression, or distress? Think about the impact on our bodies! When we realize we're only hurting ourselves, that's a scary thought.

Some people may feel that their experiences with the Catholic Church have not only made them pull away from the church but they're making them emotionally sick. This can be true for some people, but we have a choice. We have the choice to stay angry or not. We have the choice to ask God to help us to forgive. We have the choice to process this in a way that we can be emotionally and spiritually well. It's not easy. Not only can the act of forgiveness benefit us emotionally and spiritually, but studies have also found that forgiveness can benefit our physical health by "lowering the risk of heart attack, improving cholesterol levels and sleep, reducing pain, blood pressure, and levels of anxiety, depression, and stress. Research also points to an increase in the forgiveness-health connection as you age."[19]

Isn't this wonderful news that when harm has been done to us, we have the ability to improve our health just by forgiving? We can live our best lives today regardless of what is happening around us. We can do it! I've seen many people in my career do it, and we can do it too!

Just as God has forgiven us with His redeeming grace, he calls us to extend grace and forgiveness to others. Forgiving one another is very difficult on our own, but "everything is possible for the person who believes" (Matt 19:26). God's grace allows us to do things that are not possible in our human strength. Grace allows us to forgive others, which is what Jesus calls us to do.

PRAYER: "Lord God, we know with your help all things are possible. Please help us to release any anger, bitterness, or resentment that we feel and forgive the people who have hurt us so we can live our most abundant lives."

VERSE: *"Be kind and compassionate to one another, forgiving each other, just as in Christ God has forgiven you" (Eph 4:32).*

Regaining Trust & Moving Forward

"But those who hope in the Lord will renew their strength. They will soar on wings like eagles; they will run and not grow weary, they will walk and not be faint" (Isa 40:31).

When we've been betrayed, regaining trust is a process. We can't just wave a magic wand and instantly restore trust in a person, organization, or institution that has betrayed us. I believe this is why so many people have stayed away from the Catholic faith. God loves us and wants us to be able to move on from any disappointment or hurt we've experienced through the institution of the Catholic Church, or the people representing the Church. People will always disappoint us. This will never change until the end of time because we are imperfect. The truth, though, is that God will never let us down. If we trust in God's goodness and provision, and leave the how to Him, we can find our way back. God's Word says, "But blessed is the one who trusts in the LORD, whose confidence is in him" (Jer 17:7).

Regaining trust and moving forward after any betrayal or human disappointment requires time and effort. It requires a conversion and change from within. It involves a healing of the heart and a decision to forgive. As mentioned earlier, we can decide to forgive or not, and it's much healthier to forgive.

When we forgive, it doesn't mean that what the person or institution did was acceptable. It doesn't mean that we are justifying the action. On the contrary, often, when we have been hurt or betrayed, the action causing that feeling was not acceptable, moral, or righteous. It was likely human sin causing the pain.

Remember, granting forgiveness for harm is about pleasing God, not man. As we seek to forgive, regain trust, and renew our faith and love for the Church, it's important we do this because we feel it's the right thing to do, not because someone is telling us to do it. Do you feel an emptiness or loneliness within that nothing on earth has been able to quench? Do you think God is calling you to heal in some way, trust in His love, or renew your faith?

In order to move forward in the life of our parish and faith community, it's important to remember that our reasons for being Catholic must come from within our hearts. They cannot be tied to external changing circumstances, such as a certain priest, parish, or Mom's group that might eventually disband. Church ministries and events may change or stop over time. Church buildings may close and merge with other parishes. Traditions may change depending on who is in charge.

Of course, all these people, places, resources, supports, and practices are wonderful gifts from God to nurture faith and build His kingdom here on earth. It is beautiful that these things make a difference in one's life and have the power to inspire, uplift, empower, and transform our lives. But there is no guarantee they will last. Being resilient is key, and as one thing ends, we must find a way to start anew and find the next thing to support our faith, never losing sight of the real reason for our faith, which is Jesus Christ, our Savior. These other things are good and help us on our journey, but they are not the "be-all, end-all."

God gives us each other and our spiritual gifts to lift one another up, but if our faith is not connected to the heart of Jesus Christ in a profound way, we will backslide or crumble every time worldly circumstances change on our faith journey.

PRAYER: "Lord God, as we move forward from the pain and disappointments we have experienced, help us to put our trust in you. Help us move forward one step at a time and experience hope and healing in your presence and promises."

VERSE: *"For I know the plans I have for you,' declares the Lord, 'plans to prosper you and not to harm you, plans to give you hope and a future'" (Jer 29:11).*

4

A Beautiful Faith

> *"Now to him who is able to do immeasurably more than all we ask or imagine, according to his power that is at work within us, to him be glory in the church and in Christ Jesus throughout all generations, for ever and ever! Amen" (Eph 3:20-21).*

Removing the Cloud of Darkness

Aside from the pain, separation, and disillusionment caused by the sins of the clergy and the poor decisions of leaders to cover up the sins, there are other reasons Catholicism has a dark cloud over it. There are many reasons people have fallen away from the Catholic faith. Then, there are others who have chosen to stay but feel guilty because they do not believe all the doctrines or teachings. I empathize. The doctrines and teachings of the Church are not easy to understand or accept.

Let's take a look at some examples of situations that have made people feel ostracized from the Church:

• I have a dear friend whose father committed suicide four decades ago. At that excruciatingly painful time of loss, she was told by the deacon that her father would never be going to heaven. What a horrific thing to tell a teenager who just lost her father. Sadly, she has had to live with this thought even though Catholic.com asserts that people who take their lives are not necessarily committing a mortal sin because psychological factors can impede their knowledge and consent of the act.[20] Thankfully, in the early 90s, the Church realized that mental health plays a part in this tragic situation, and the Catechism was revised accordingly. It is imperative that faith formation programs and catechists are kept up to date with such teachings because in 2010, elementary and middle school students I know were still being taught that suicide is a sin.

• A devout Catholic woman felt bullied into leaving a women's church group after she expressed her concern for women who have been raped and the church's staunch stance on abortion. The idea that women do not have a choice is challenging for many to wrap their heads around. I do believe in the right to life and the sanctity of all human life. It's in the instance of rape that the teaching can appear insensitive and inhumane. After researching, I discovered in the case of rape, the Ethical and Religious Directives for Catholic Health Care Services allow for emergency contraception if fertilization has not yet occurred.[21] Why are we not making this publicly known? For many, the Catholic Church can appear rigid, inhumane, and heartless. Perhaps through compassionate proactive public education and making information like this known, more women would have this knowledge and take action quicker in the instance of rape to ensure conception does not occur. Perhaps by humanizing the messaging, women would be more open and receptive to hearing all of the positive life-giving reasons and options rather than continuing to be reminded of what they should not do.

- Members of the LGBTQ+ community feel targeted and ostracized from many (if not most) of the Catholic and Christian communities in which they live. There are countless stories of these people being denied services by Catholic or Christian organizations and business owners. Church reform could include a more inclusive understanding of LGBTQ+ issues and how members of the Church can engage with these community members with greater compassion, focusing on the dignity and worth of every individual as created in the image of God. This aligns with the Catholic Church's teaching that all people are indeed created in the image of God, which affirms their dignity and calls for respect and love towards every individual.[22] The Catechism of the Catholic Church also teaches that "They must be accepted with respect, compassion and sensitivity."[23]

- A divorced woman, unable to attain a marriage annulment, was ostracized from the Church many years ago. She is hurt and bitter. She longs for a reunion with her faith but is not sure she feels welcome to return to the Catholic Church. Fortunately, the Church's process for an annulment was streamlined when the Code of Canon Law was revised in 1983. The process was further streamlined in 2015, with *Mitis iudex*,[24] making the process more accessible and merciful, showing compassion and understanding towards individuals in difficult marital situations. Thankfully, divorced persons without an annulment can still participate in the sacramental life of their parish. I wonder if she knows this?

There are other reasons people feel ostracized, have left the Church, or disagree with its teachings. Some people believe we should not pray for the intercession of Mary or the Saints. Others have a hard time believing that the Eucharist is truly the body, blood, soul, and divinity of Jesus Christ. Some don't want to confess their sins to a priest in the sacrament of Reconciliation. Maybe Mass is too boring, or there isn't a fun community gathering after each service. Many feel there are too many rules to live up to or that Catholics place rules and doctrine before the love of neighbor. Others have had a poor experience with a religious or lay member of the Church. All of these reasons are real. We cannot discount people's feelings and emotions, many of which are tied to their beliefs and past experiences. We must find a way to bridge the gap and welcome them home.

Catholicism is not easy, nor is it meant to be. Some of the most rewarding things in life—such as a strong marriage, a college degree, regular exercise, and healthy eating—require dedication, commitment, and intentional effort. When we neglect these efforts, the results reflect our lack of input, leading to challenges like marital struggles, failed courses, weight gain, and declining health. Similarly, with perseverance and an open and sincere heart, Catholicism can be a beautiful journey that offers moral guidance and theological structure, helping us grow in union with God (and let's face it, we all need rules and structure!). This is not a journey we can embark on alone though. Only through God's grace and total reliance on Him can we achieve salvation and overcome our fallen ways, preparing us to one day enjoy eternal life in heaven.

PRAYER: "Lord Jesus, help us to see the beauty of the Catholic faith. Show us how to pray more fervently and seek the guidance of the Holy Spirit to persevere in growing our faith within a community of believers."

VERSE: "Blessed is the one who perseveres under trial because, having stood the test, that person will receive the crown of life that the Lord has promised to those who love him" (James 1:12).

Misconceptions in the Catholic Faith

Archbishop Fulton J. Sheen once said, "There are not one hundred people in the United States who hate the Catholic Church, but there are millions who hate what they wrongly perceive the Catholic Church to be."[25]

Many beautiful aspects of the Catholic faith are misunderstood. Several of these beliefs and traditions of the faith set Catholicism apart in a unique way from other Christian denominations. Biblical scholars and theologians have written plenty of books and apologetics on these topics. I'm not a biblical scholar or a theologian. I'm an ordinary Cradle Catholic who desires to know and understand my faith better and help others to appreciate the beauty and richness of the faith. I am offering my exploration of the following seven topics: Mary, Saints, Reconciliation, Mass, Holy Communion, One True Church, and Faith plus Works.

1. Mary

Many people who oppose Catholic teachings feel that there is an overemphasis on Mary and less emphasis on Jesus. I agree that there is a dominant focus and reverence for Mary, but the good news is that it all points to her son, our Savior, Jesus Christ. None of what Catholics believe is meant to take away from Jesus, our redeemer and Savior of the world.

Unfortunately, there is such a variation in the way Catholic communities, parishes, and individuals practice their faith that it makes it very possible that some Catholics inadvertently or overtly focus more on Mary than Jesus. They may lose sight of the fact that Jesus is our Savior, not Mary. Many Catholics still believe and say that we pray "to" Mary, but a canon lawyer priest, who advised me with this book, assured me that this is incorrect. Paragraphs 2673-2676 in the Catechism of the Catholic Church clarify that Catholics honor Mary and seek her intercession, but the ultimate prayer and worship are directed to God alone.[26]

That said, without Mary, we would have no Jesus and no Savior. Mary was and is essential to Jesus as His mother. Mary is an intercessor who advocates and goes straight to Jesus with our prayers. Mary's intercessory power comes directly from Jesus. He is not jealous when we go to His mother asking for her prayers; He is honored and pleased!

Here's a renewed way to look at Mary. She is our spiritual mother and the mother of our Universal Church. God gives us sweet Mary, the mother of Jesus, a virgin betrothed without sin, as someone to emulate and look up to as a role model who lived a saintly, holy life."The angel went to her and said, "Greetings, you who are highly favored! The Lord is with you" (Luke 1:28). As Christians, we can strive to emulate Mary in our words and actions. She is a beautiful example of purity and goodness.

Can you imagine how scared Mary was when the angel Gabriel came to her? The Bible tells us that she had no relations with a man yet would conceive and bear a son. "The angel answered, 'The Holy Spirit will come on you, and the power of the Most High will overshadow you. So the holy one to be born will be called the Son of God'" (Luke 1:35). Mary gave her "yes" to God so willingly. Will we do the same? Will we give our life to God and put our faith and trust in Him? Mary is ever-present to help us draw closer to her son, Jesus.

There is documentation of the miraculous power of Mary through her son, Jesus Christ. Just as the apostles had the intercessory power to perform miracles through Jesus, so does Mary. It makes sense that if Jesus gave the apostles this gift, He would also give His mother, Mary, this grace as well. Nine approved Marian apparitions are documented and three possess historical and spiritual scrutiny. Since 1858, over 7,000 miraculous cures have been reported by Our Lady of

Lourdes pilgrims, with 70 cases being deemed scientifically inexplicable, meeting the standards of a "miracle" by the Lourdes Medical Bureau. You can read more about this at www.magiscenter.com.[27] You see, Mary is not just a woman in the Bible. She is the mother of Jesus Christ, our Savior. She is seated at the right hand of God as Queen of Heaven and Earth. Mary is a beautiful gift from God that is to be cherished.

2. Saints

According to the United States Conference of Catholic Bishops, "All Christians are called to be Saints. Saints are persons in heaven (officially canonized or not) who lived heroically virtuous lives, offered their lives for others, were martyred for the faith, and are worthy of imitation."[28]

Most people don't rebuke the idea that saints were tremendously holy people of God who deserve to be elevated because of their faithful servanthood. The part that is difficult for many (non-Catholics and protestants) to understand is the idea of praying for the saints to intercede on our behalf. I can understand the confusion and reasoning that we should only honor Jesus. However, walk with me on this journey...

Imagine for a moment Jesus in heaven. Do you imagine He will be alone? Or do you imagine that He will be surrounded by angels and saints? Why wouldn't someone as important as Jesus, the Savior of the world, not have an army of saints and angels surrounding Him and leading the charge along with Him? God gives us each of these spiritual warriors to support us, to provide us with guidance and hope, and to intercede on our behalf, taking our intentions straight to God.

Have you ever asked someone to pray for you? Perhaps you asked for prayers for a loved one or family member who was sick. Asking the saints to pray for us is the same thing. We believe they are alive in heaven and can intercede for us just like those here on earth. In either case, whether we ask people on earth to pray for us or saints in heaven to pray for us, it's important to note that the power comes from God, not the person or saint themselves.

The saints were sinners like you and I. They were real people who walked this earth, with strengths and weaknesses, virtues and vices. There is likely a saint that each one of us can relate to and learn from in some way. It doesn't mean we worship them. On the contrary, we look up to them for their goodness, their saintly life, the miracles they performed, and even how they overcame adversity. They are present to help us draw nearer to God and to live more saintly lives ourselves."Their responsibility is to equip God's people to do his work and build up the church, the body of Christ." (Eph 4:12 NLT).

Many Catholics dedicate time to intercessory prayer, asking a specific saint to intercede and pray with us to our heavenly Father on behalf of a particular cause. The prayer to St. Michael the Archangel is a beautiful prayer asking this saint to help defend us in battle against the wickedness and snares of the devil. Interestingly, in 1884, Pope Leo XIII requested that the St. Michael prayer be prayed at the end of Catholic Masses worldwide.[29] Recently, the parishioners at my church started saying this prayer at the end of every Mass, too. It is beautiful.

St. Jude Thaddeus is the patron saint of miracles and lost causes. I had a client in my coaching practice who prayed for the intercession of St. Jude for healing with fear. St. Anthony of Padua is the patron saint of lost items and is an excellent example of humility and gentleness, offering encouragement to unmarried women, the less fortunate, expectant mothers, and infertile women. I recall praying for the intercession of St. Anthony to help find lost items as a child, and we always found them! St. Francis of Assisi is the patron saint of animals, and many ask for his intercession on behalf of sick pets and animals.[30]

My mother-in-law suffered a life-threatening illness with a high fever as a small child. Her loved ones prayed for St. Rocco's intercession. She believes God healed her through the intercession of this saint. Believing in the intercessory power of the saints is a beautiful way for Catholics to relate to other saintly people in their suffering and healing and to draw us closer to a trusting relationship with God.

Everything in Catholicism- Mary, the Saints, the Mass, the Sacraments, Holy Communion- all points to Jesus. It's not about worshiping anything or anyone other than Jesus. He gives us this support as a part of His spiritual army. We can pray directly to Jesus, of course! I don't think we need Mary or the saints to have an excellent Christian faith; otherwise, only Catholics would be going to heaven, and that is a ludicrous thought. They are a beautiful aspect of the Catholic faith that elevates the importance of Jesus as our Savior. God doesn't go it alone, and He gives us many supports, mentors, and prayer warriors to help us through this challenging life and guide us in our journey to living a virtuous life. What a blessing and gift!

3. Reconciliation

Many people question the Catholic practice of Reconciliation. They question whether confessing one's sins to a priest is necessary. They ask, why can't I go directly to God with my sins? These are all great questions.

First of all, we can go to God with anything, for it is God who ultimately forgives and heals us of our sins. That being said, I have experienced a deep transformation within myself through the Sacrament of Reconciliation. There is something very profound about sharing our deepest regrets and failings out loud in the presence of a priest and our desire to be transformed through the power of the Holy Spirit in our thoughts, words, and actions. This outward public activity is both humbling and empowering.

My good friend Fred shared with me two reasons, in layman's terms, why Catholics believe confession to a priest is beneficial. First, confession to a priest serves as a visible witness to our community that we have sinned against God and against man. Second, the priest can give us wise counsel and help us achieve lasting repentance for our sins.

Beyond these benefits, there is evidence of the need for vocal confession in John 20:23, where the Lord gives the Apostles two options-to forgive or retain- thus establishing them as merciful judges. It can be argued that they would not know which to forgive and which to retain if there wasn't a verbal confession of sin and display of contrition.

In addition, after Jesus' resurrection, He tells the apostles to follow His example and receive the Holy Spirit, giving them the power to absolve people's sins, which is what the priest does in the Sacrament of Confession. The priest receives the sin through the sacrament, but it is Jesus who forgives the sin. God's Word says, "Confess your sins to one another and pray for one another, that you may be healed. The prayer of a righteous person has great power as it is working" (James 5:16 KJV). Catholic priests can trace their ordinations back to the apostles. This is called apostolic succession. This is evidence that Jesus instituted the Sacrament of Reconciliation, which is how He desires for us to confess our sins.

Going to Reconciliation (Confession) is an uncomfortable thing for sure. I get it. If you recall at the beginning of this book, I shared some very unpleasant experiences. Despite that, I can tell you that I've also had dozens of positive experiences where I have felt spiritual cleansing in a real and profound way. I still get nervous about going to Reconciliation to this day. I still sometimes wonder if I'm doing it right. I sometimes still question if I'm truly forgiven. It takes work to have faith. It's not easy, but I now understand that it grieves God when we don't believe in and accept His forgiveness, as it discounts the magnitude and power of His saving grace and His genuine love to heal us.

What I've learned to believe is that I'm truly speaking to God through the priest. When I do that, the fear diminishes, and I let my heart take over. I try to speak from my heart and share sorrow and repentance for my sins.

God's Word instructs us that holding on to sin prevents us from prospering in God's peace and joy. "Whoever conceals their sins does not prosper, but the one who confesses and renounces them finds mercy" (Prov 28:13 NIV). Confession cleanses our hearts of our sins and reconciles us with God's love and forgiveness. I heard Mother Angelica once say that Confession is "like taking a bath for our soul." What a beautiful description. We definitely wouldn't refrain from taking a bath for months or even years. As our body needs to be cleansed, our spiritual self and soul must also be cleansed.

The Sacrament of Confession is not an easy aspect of the Catholic faith, but it is a beautiful gift to be experienced. "If we confess our sins, he is faithful and just and will forgive us our sins and purify us from all unrighteousness" (1 John 1:9). It can help us to live a more holy and saintly life and bring us peace as we journey closer to Jesus' good, pleasing, and perfect will for our lives.

4. Mass

If we're not engaged and seeking to learn and be spiritually fed, Mass can be boring. Being open to one "a-ha" moment at each Mass where we feel God is speaking directly to us can help considerably to make Mass a more meaningful experience. We have to be open, ready, and have a willing heart. It's not easy. Our minds can get distracted. We can get lazy and not go to Mass when we don't "feel" like it or when our busy lives and other commitments take priority. I heard Matthew Kelly (international speaker, author, and founder of Dynamic Catholic Institute) once say, "We do not judge an activity by how we feel before we do it; we judge it by how we feel after we do it." I love that!

This is a gross oversimplification and perhaps a poor comparison but think about exercise, chores, doing laundry, going to work, and a multitude of other things that we might not "feel" like doing but know they're the right thing to do. If we only do what we "feel" like doing, we'll be a disaster. More importantly, think about how you feel after you accomplish something like doing the laundry, making a special dinner, reading a book, exercising, or eating healthy. Going to Mass is no different. We may not want to go, but when we open ourselves to Jesus present in the Holy Eucharist, He fills us up in more ways than we could ever imagine.

The reason Catholics go to Mass isn't primarily to "get something out of it," though. Yes, the Eucharist is spiritual food for our souls and our lives, but the primary purpose of Mass is to give thanks to the Lord for all He has done for us and give our praise to God as individuals and as a community. Attending Mass with a heart of gratitude to God for all of His blessings and engaging in heartfelt prayer and worship makes the experience that much more meaningful, and opens our hearts to His love and grace.

Some people claim that Catholics don't teach and focus enough on the gospel message of Jesus. The great news and truth of the matter is that 89.8 percent of the Gospels and 71.5 percent of the entire New Testament are covered in the Sunday and weekday lectionaries over a three-year period, according to Fr. Felix Just, S.J., as reported by Catholic Answers.[31] The truth is that Catholics revere and hold the gospel message in a place of honor during the Mass!

Perhaps Catholics have not always practiced the faith as if the Bible is the living, breathing Word of God, or it may not appear that way. I, for one, can testify to the strength and power in memorizing and believing the promises of God in the Holy Bible. God's Word is a "lamp to my feet and a light for my path" (Ps 119:105, NKJV). The Scriptures give us every instruction on living a good, holy, and righteous life. I would never go a day again in my life without studying or reflecting on at least one verse from the Holy Bible. It breathes life, goodness, wisdom, and peace into every aspect of my life. Three terrific Bible verses that highlight the vital role of Scripture in our lives and Eucharistic celebrations are:

- "All Scripture is given by inspiration of God, and is profitable for doctrine, for reproof, for correction, for instruction in righteousness, that the man of God may be complete, thoroughly equipped for every good work" (2 Tim 3:16-17).
- "But he said, 'Blessed rather are those who hear the word of God and keep it!'" (Luke 11:28).
- "But he answered, 'It is written, "Man shall not live by bread alone, but by every word that comes from the mouth of God"'" (Matt 4:4).

In addition to hearing Scripture, the Mass is a beautiful, holy celebration of the Eucharist, where we commemorate the sacrifice Jesus made on the cross for our sins. "This is my body, which is given for you. Do this in remembrance of me" (Luke 22:19 NLT). Think about it…we experience the living presence of God in every Mass! What a beautiful, priceless gift waiting for us to experience. Celebrating each Mass with a grateful heart of love, devotion, and thanksgiving makes this gift an even more beautiful, joy-filled experience.

5. Holy Communion

The Eucharist is central to the Catholic Christian life, where bread and wine become the body and blood of Christ during Mass. This change is called transubstantiation.[32] Unfortunately, and depending on the survey results we read, between 56-69% of Catholics do not believe that Jesus' body and blood are truly present in the Eucharist. This means that only about 30% believe in the real presence of Jesus in the Eucharist. This statistic has been confirmed in a Catholicexchange.com article titled "Nine Proofs of the True Presence."[33] According to this article, that percentage only increases to 62% for practicing Catholics. I understand. It's definitely a difficult concept and belief to grasp. If you're a person with a more scientific mind or who likes "proof," it can be doubly challenging to wholeheartedly believe that this is true.

I would even dare to say it's not a person's fault if they don't believe it yet. The Catholic Church can do a better job with the education piece. Of course, we're not entirely off the hook. We need to take the initiative to invest the time to learn about these things. I'll admit that, until recently, I was on the fence about this myself. In defense of the Church, I have seen considerable efforts more recently to help people believe that the Eucharist is the real presence. Things like faith formation talks, apologetics speakers, and informational resources placed in the back of the church have been valuable resources at my parish.

For the scientific folk, there is proof one might find very interesting. According to this same article in catholicexchange.com, there have been well over 100 Church-approved Eucharistic miracles dating back to the early Middle Ages. In recent decades, a dozen Eucharistic miracles have occurred throughout the world. Samples have been taken from Eucharist hosts and studied in scientific laboratories. One such miracle happened in the parish of St. Anthony of Padua in Sokolka, Poland, in 2008 when a host that was dropped during communion was put in water per Church protocol. It was safely locked in the sacristy.

A week later, the priest opened the safe to dispose of the dissolved host properly. He was amazed to see the host intact. The appearance of the host had changed, with the very center of the host being a bloody fleshy substance. The bishop decided to have two world-renowned forensic laboratories determine the contents of the host. Each specimen contained a piece of the inner bloody fleshy substance as well as the outer rim of the intact host. Unaware of each other's study, both laboratories found identical results. The independent findings determined it was heart tissue from a person severely beaten on the chest, as Jesus was. The blood type was AB+, the same blood type that has been found in every other Eucharistic miracle. Additionally, this is the same blood type found on the Shroud of Turin and the Sudarium (the burial cloths of Jesus as in John 20:6-7). Only 5% of the population has this blood type. Further remarkable evidence is that the heart tissue was alive, an extraordinary circumstance considering that human tissue cannot survive outside the body for more than 20 minutes.[34]

Holy Communion is one of the most beautiful aspects of the Catholic Church. What a gift to have the opportunity to receive the body, blood, soul, and divinity of Jesus Christ in the Eucharistic Celebration of Mass on any given day of the week. "So Jesus said again, 'I tell you the truth, unless you eat the flesh of the Son of Man and drink his blood, you cannot have eternal life within you. But anyone who eats my flesh and drinks my blood has eternal life, and I will raise that person on the last day. For my flesh is true food, and my blood is true drink. Anyone who eats my flesh and drinks my blood remains in me, and I in him'" (John 6:53-56). After Jesus said this, many left because they could not accept this teaching. He didn't say, "Wait, come back; I only meant that figuratively." He asked the apostles, "Are you also going to leave?" Simon Peter responded, "Lord, to whom would we go? You have the words that give eternal life" (John 6:67-68). As we reflect on this, may it draw us closer to Jesus, present in the Eucharist, our one true and trustworthy source of eternal life.

6. One True Church

Catholicism's claim to be the "one true church" is often misunderstood and can be a source of division between Catholics and members of other Christian denominations. There is a lack of understanding among Catholics themselves as well. Does "one true church" mean that all other forms of Christianity are false? Does it mean that the Catholic Church is the only church recognized by God or does it mean that the Catholic Church holds all the truths that other religions do not? These ideas can be confusing and divisive.

So what does "one true church" really mean? The best description I've found was in an article by Deacon Pedro called "Deacon-structing the One, True Church." He states that Christ established only one Church as a "visible and spiritual community" and that this one Church subsists in the Catholic Church.[35] This Church is governed by the successor of Peter (the Pope) and the Bishops in communion with him.

Deacon Pedro continues to explain that the key word in understanding this concept lies in the word "subsist" which, according to the Oxford Dictionary, means "to exist or continue to exist; to keep alive."[36] He continues to say that "in this sense, the Church of Christ, 'continues to exist, or keeps herself alive' in the Catholic Church...To say that the Church of Christ subsists in the Catholic Church is very different from saying that the Church of Christ is the Catholic Church."[37]

This explanation makes a lot more sense to me in terms of how Catholicism fits into the roots of Christianity. The elements of the Church that Christ founded over 2,000 years ago can still be found and exist within the Catholic Church. Catholicism has roots that go back to Peter, as described in Matthew 16:18, which declares, "Now I say to you that you are Peter (which means 'rock'), and upon this rock I will build my church, and all the powers of hell will not conquer it." According to an article by RCSpirituality, "He (Christ) appointed Peter as the rock on which the Church was built. The Pope is the successor of Peter."[38]

In an effort to unite and build bridges among denominations, my question is, "Can Catholics believe they participate in the "one true church" that is the best and most "complete" of all the other denominations and still welcome all those they meet with a humble heart of acceptance? In our human weakness it seems tough to do if one believes he/she has something "better than" any other faith. Catholicism may be the most "complete" faith, but God calls us to be humble and love and embrace everyone, even atheists, and we must find a way to do this. Catholics have to be careful not to pompously project arrogance when speaking of their faith, as I have witnessed. We must look at everyone as a precious child of God and pray for their salvation. Being an example of Christ, loving others, and praying for them is the very best thing we can do as Catholics and Christians.

I hope we can all agree that God came to save ALL people, not just Catholics. "For this is how God loved the world: He gave his one and only Son, so that everyone who believes in him will not perish but have eternal life" (John 3:16).

It is reassuring that Christ's first Church exists within and is carried on by the Catholic Church. There is no reason to believe that other Christian denominations are not also keeping aspects of the Church of Christ alive in this world. I think we need to be open to learning and growing in our faith as one Universal church in the world.

We can learn from other Christians who have such a deep devotion and love for God. Catholics shouldn't feel threatened by them, as I have witnessed over and over in my journey as a Catholic Christian. While theological and doctrinal differences do exist, we are one in unity and love for Christ.[39] My sister and several close friends are Protestant and one of my dearest friends is Baptist. Their faith is beautiful, and I've learned more about praising and worshiping God from them than most of my Catholic influences. I admire them immensely for their faith, surrendering their lives fully to God, and accepting Jesus as their personal Savior. I can't imagine upon their death God saying, "Well, you're not Catholic, so I'm not granting you entrance into heaven." God might be more likely to say to a Catholic, "Well, you have 'said' your prayers, but you have not 'prayed' them or given your life and heart fully to Jesus as your Savior." This certainly gives us something to think about.

Jesus gives us clear instructions on getting to heaven. "I am the way, the truth, and the life. No one can come to the Father except through me" (John 14:6 NKJV). God's Word is clear that the only way to heaven is through Jesus. As Catholics and Christians, it's essential to accept all of God's children and believe in their ability to get to heaven if they commit their lives and hearts to Jesus. All people of all religions are loved equally by God, and while there are differences in how faith is practiced, no person is "better than" anyone else because of their religious affiliation. When we don't believe this, we are automatically creating a schism, a separation, a hierarchy that grieves God. My concern is that, as Catholics, we have elevated ourselves to a place above others, especially with such an unclear understanding of our belief that we are the "one true church." I hope Church leaders will do a better job of clarifying such beliefs and that, with God's grace, greater unity and respect among religions and all of God's people will continue to happen.

7. Faith Plus Works

Catholics believe in the importance of both faith and works. I don't doubt that faith alone - as Protestant Christians believe - could and likely would grant someone the gift of salvation. I also feel that we can't just say a sinner's prayer and accept Jesus as our Lord and Savior and then be saved without putting those words into action with a heartfelt desire to know, love, and please God.

In the pursuit of Christian unity and in an effort to overcome the historical divisions stemming from the Reformation, it's helpful to know that the Catholic Church and Lutheran World Federation came together in 1999, affirming that justification (how individuals are made right with God) is by God's grace alone through faith in Jesus Christ. Both denominations are one in the belief that faith involves a transformative relationship with God rather than a passive acceptance and that the beauty of God's grace manifests itself in our lives as faith and works. Feel free to read the 1999 joint declaration of the doctrine of justification for more information.[40]

God's grace, in action, manifests itself in a beautiful way through the lives of many Catholics. The Catholic Church has a longstanding reputation for helping the poor and those in need. According to CatholicCharitiesUSA.org, "In 2022, the Catholic Charities network, covering the United States and five territories, served more than 15 million people in need at more than 3,900 network sites."[41] In addition to Catholic Charities, many other Catholic organizations exist to help the most vulnerable people in our world. Such organizations include Caritas Internationalis, Catholic Relief Services (CRS), Society of St. Vincent de Paul, Maryknoll Missionaries, Aid to the Church in Need (ACN), Missionaries of Charity, Jesuit Refugee Service (JRS), Catholic Medical Mission Board (CMMB), Cross Catholic Outreach, Knights of Columbus, Food for the Poor, Catholic Worker Movement, and Salesian Missions. Collectively, these Catholic organizations are estimated to serve the needs of hundreds of millions of people worldwide each year.[42]

God's Word says: "Suppose a brother or a sister is without clothes and daily food. If one of you says to them, 'Go in peace; keep warm and well fed,' but does nothing about their physical needs, what good is it? In the same way, faith by itself, if it is not accompanied by action, is dead" (James 2:15-17 NIV).

Scripture instructs us not just to use our words but to actually help people and serve them as much as we can. "Dear children, let us not love with words or speech but with actions and in truth" (1 John 3:18). "Truly I tell you, whatever you did for one of the least of these brothers and sisters of mine, you did for me" (Matt 25:40).

Serving the needs of others- the poor, the marginalized, and the needy- is most rewarding when done with a joyful heart rather than out of obligation or guilt, as I have seen happen. Other Christians sometimes feel that Catholics think they can "work" their way into heaven. This is not what Catholics believe and should not be the spirit in which Catholics serve the needs of others. These are acts of service that imitate Christ and cause us to be a light to this world. Bringing Christ's love, hope, and healing to the forgotten and hopeless cannot grant us everlasting life alone, but in combination with our faith in Jesus as our Lord and Savior, it can show us what true discipleship really means.

"For I was hungry and you gave me something to eat, I was thirsty and you gave me something to drink, I was a stranger and you invited me in, I needed clothes and you clothed me, I was sick and you looked after me, I was in prison and you came to visit me" (Matthew 25:35–36).

In conclusion, while there are misconceptions surrounding the Catholic teachings and practices regarding Mary and the Saints, sacraments such as Reconciliation and Eucharist, the Mass, and the ecclesiastical positions of "one true church" and faith plus works, these are beautiful aspects of the Catholic faith and tradition. Growing our faith through these beliefs and other practices within the Church is a gift God gives us. He knows how easy it is to slip away from our faith, especially with the distractions of the secular world. Catholicism may not be easy, but the consequences of losing our faith are devastating to our lives and our souls.

When we are growing in faith, trusting in God, and accepting Jesus as our Savior, we have continual hope in our future and the promise of everlasting life. When we're not growing in faith and being fed through the Mass, prayer, Scripture, a community of believers, and the sacraments, evil can creep in, leading to discouragement, loneliness, and hopelessness.

The Catholic Church provides a comprehensive array of supports to help us move toward God's holy and perfect will for our lives as He utilizes us to build His kingdom here on earth. I heard it once said that "Catholicism is the gift that everyone needs." It is a beautiful gift that can look intimidating, but when opened and utilized, it is the brightest, most rewarding gift imaginable.

Community

One of the strengths of the Catholic Church is the presence of a very supportive community of believers. Through a community of believers, we can be supported personally and spiritually. As I previously mentioned, by participating in groups such as faith sharing, Bible study, Daughters of Mary, the Seven Sisters Apostolate, Christ Renews His Parish Welcome retreat, mission, and religious studies, we can truly experience being one body in Christ.

Investing the time to continue my spiritual growth in my adult years has made all the difference for me since my early years as a Catholic. Those faith formation activities, along with reading Scripture and devotionals, increasing my prayer time, participating in Eucharistic adoration, listening to Christian music, and attending Mass more regularly, have helped my faith and love for God to blossom and grow deeper.

Take it one step at a time. What is one manageable thing you feel you could do this week to nurture your faith and sense of community?

PRAYER: "Lord Jesus, thank you for the gift of the Catholic Church and Godly family, friends, and sisters and brothers in Christ who can lift us up and support us in our faith journeys. Thank you for the gift of community activities that build our faith. Please help us to seek them out and open doors that will bring Godly people and activities into our lives. Amen."

VERSE: "For as in one body we have many members, and the members do not all have the same function, so we, though many, are one body in Christ, and individually members one of another" (Rom 12:4-5 KJV).

Continuing Education

Members of the Catholic Church need continuing education in order to understand the Church's teachings and accept them more fully. We don't just believe what we believe because someone tells us to believe it. Forming beliefs, from receiving information to acceptance as truth, is a process. According to research by Connors, M. H., & Halligan, P. W. (2022), "Beliefs are convictions about what we accept as true. They provide the fundamental framework that we use to understand and engage meaningfully with the world." These researchers suggest a 5 stage cognitive model of belief formation. The first step is moving from a precursor to the belief. Second, search for meaning. Third, evaluation of the belief. Fourth, acceptance of the belief. Fifth, the effects of the belief.[43] Despite this, there is no absolute or automatic guarantee that the information will be believed.

Beliefs are a journey of the heart, not just the mind. This process is not a straight line. We should exercise gentleness and grace with ourselves and others on this journey of faith. Build one another up. Listen to hear, empathize, and understand. Gently share resources that have helped you. Don't tell them they are wrong in what they think and believe. We think we are helping, but remember, we are human beings with feelings. Yes, it's pride that gets hurt, but we are all prideful people and nobody likes to be told what to think or believe. In fact, beliefs don't work that way at all. We believe what we believe not only because something has entered our minds, but it has also entered our hearts. This is not only a mindset change; this is a heart change. It takes time. It's not something we can hear once, and we automatically believe it. It must first start with education and increased knowledge of the doctrine and teaching of the Church. It must be presented with gentleness, compassion, and love. No, it shouldn't be sugar-coated, but it should include what the Catholic Church teaches and why. The why should consist of the reasons and justification for the teaching in a simplistic, easy-to-understand manner. It has to reach the heart and not only the mind. The only way we can shift our beliefs is through a shift in our hearts, and it starts with education and planting seeds of God's wisdom and grace.

So, where do we go from here? How can we help Catholics to better understand and believe the doctrine and teachings of the Church? What if priests and deacons talked about one fact in question during every Mass? What about launching a television campaign to build a better understanding and appreciation of Catholicism for all people? What if these messages spoke to the miracles of Jesus through the intercession of the saints, the beauty of the Sacraments, or why Catholics believe in honoring (not worshiping) Mary? Perhaps we should not need evidence or explanations in order to believe and have faith, but the reality is that there are so many forces opposing Catholicism and Christianity. In our world today, we need to use the facts that we have about Jesus' life, the miracles he performed, the miracles that are happening through His mother, Mary, to shout to the world that we have a Savior.

Continuing education is a critical piece of the puzzle, and the lack of it is one of the primary reasons Catholics and non-Catholics do not understand the teachings and doctrine of the Church. I pray that Church leaders and clergy will make a concerted effort to educate people on Catholic tradition and beliefs and why Catholics believe what we believe. I am encouraged by the more recent faith formation activities at my parish. We are moving in the right direction, and it brings such hope! To continue to grow in the knowledge and love of Christ, as well as Catholic Church teaching, it is important that we also take an active role in learning about our faith. The Catechism of the Catholic Church is an excellent resource for reliable answers. In addition, with the plethora of online resources available, there is never a shortage of places to find the answers to questions we may have.

PRAYER: "*Lord God, thank you for the opportunity to practice our beautiful faith within a community of parishes. Thank you for the organized practices, history, teachings, and doctrine that have helped us to be the best people we can be. Help us to grow closer to you each day by earnestly continuing to learn about the practice of our faith. Amen.*"

VERSE: "*So then, just as you received Christ Jesus as Lord, continue to live your lives in him, rooted and built up in him, strengthened in the faith as you were taught, and overflowing with thankfulness*" (Col 2:6-7 NIV).

5

Love Above All

"And now these three remain: faith, hope and love. But the greatest of these is love" (1 Cor 13:13).

Love without Judgment

"Teacher, which is the greatest commandment in the Law?" Jesus replied: 'Love the Lord your God with all your heart and with all your soul and with all your mind.' This is the first and greatest commandment. And the second is like it: 'Love your neighbor as yourself.' All the Law and the Prophets hang on these two commandments" (Matt 22:36-40).

I had a huge wake-up call in my mid-30s when I learned how important it is to love without judgment. I was applying to graduate school with the intention of pursuing a Master's degree in counseling. I was the mother of three young children, and it was a big decision for me to return to school at that time in my life. I was excited about starting this new journey to fulfill God's calling and help people overcome challenges and live their best lives. This would be a dream come true.

One of the graduate school entrance requirements was to take a personality screening to make sure I was a suitable candidate for the program. After completing it, I was shocked to learn that I needed to speak with the program director because my score was below the acceptable mark. I was devastated. I thought I was a perfect candidate who would become a wonderful counselor. Come to find out, it was my strong, conservative Christian beliefs that were holding me back from being admitted into the program at this Jesuit College affiliated with the Roman Catholic Church.

It was a huge wake-up call for me when I realized how important it is to love and accept all people. I realized that it would not be professional or ethical for me to have judgmental thoughts about a student, adult, or couple coming to me with certain beliefs, feelings, and history, or about how "sinful" or "bad" they were. I did not have to deny or give up my beliefs, but rather make a commitment to build trust and respect in all of my counselor-client relationships. I couldn't let pride, judgment, or criticism enter into my therapeutic work. This was a very perplexing and soul-searching time in my life. Thankfully, after discussing the results of my assessment with the director of the program, I was admitted. I was so grateful, and from that moment on, I vowed to have an open, compassionate mind, striving to love others without judgment no matter their lifestyle, behavior, or beliefs.

So, is it possible to have strong convictions, viewpoints, and beliefs yet treat one another with an agape kind of love? The type of love that has no judgments, no pride, no defensiveness, but loves with an open heart, a heart that is willing to learn and let the Holy Spirit guide one's thoughts and actions in accordance with the Holy Spirit and the Word of God. Is this possible when someone has such strong conservative beliefs? I surely hope so, but I don't think it's something that can be achieved through our own merit. The Holy Spirit needs to be at work in our minds and our hearts. Humility is also an important part of the puzzle. If we act with pride, believing that we have the answer, the one truth, the one way, or the one religion and belief system that is better than all the rest, how can we set aside those beliefs to let other thoughts in that may deepen our relationship with Jesus and love for all people? It's a thought I've been pondering quite a bit lately. It's one that I think is important to ponder. What I'm referring to is perfect love, an agape kind of love, and a love that accepts others, no matter what.

In my mind, love and compassion ought to be the first response no matter if someone has had an abortion, gotten divorced, or is affiliated with the LGBTQ+ community. When we encounter a person experiencing a situation that is contrary to our beliefs, how do we respond? Do we think to ourselves, "What a lovely person." "That must've been a difficult situation to face." "How can I love this person at this moment?" Or, are we thinking more about what we "disapprove of" in that person? I am concerned that the behavior one views as sinful has become, for many, the primary thing thought about about rather than the beauty and goodness in this person. No matter the situation or how someone's beliefs or actions conflict with our own beliefs, I hope we will all respond with humility, love, and grace. More importantly, I believe this is the way God wants us to respond.

I don't have all the answers. I seek to come from a place of humility and, in many ways, am searching for the truth myself. My concern is that when we put doctrine, rules, and religious beliefs before the love of our brother or sister in Christ, I think we have God's plan a little backward. They have to coexist in a synergistic way. As a Catholic and Christian community, we have to wake up. We have to see that we are doing something wrong if millions of people are leaving the faith. We have to right the wrongs and forge a new era of integrity, humility, discipleship, peace, unity, and love. Our world desperately needs it. The people in our communities and families desperately need it. We need it.

As we move forward with increased love, acceptance, and tolerance for one another and all of our shortcomings, may we remember that each of us, as human beings, has different life experiences that influence how we feel, what we believe, and the decisions we make. God created every one of us unique. No two people have the same DNA. How marvelous this is, and it opens the opportunity for each of us to be wise and in tune with this fact as we interact with every other human being.

PRAYER: "Lord, help us to interact with one another in a way that seeks to understand and love rather than judge. Help us to place the love of our neighbor above all else as we imitate God's love in all we do. Amen."

VERSE: "Do everything in love" (1 Cor 16:14).

Acceptance, Tolerance, Compassion

"You must be compassionate, just as your Father is compassionate" (Luke 6:36 NLT).

Letting go of judgmental tendencies (the ones that are more harmful than helpful) is something we can change. It does take time and an intentional desire, commitment, and effort to make a personal conversion in both our minds and our hearts.

But you might be saying, "What if I believe Christians are to judge others' actions?" That is a valid question. Some Christians believe that we ought to judge, and others believe that God is the only judge. The Bible can be difficult to understand, with passages within Scripture that may appear to have conflicting messages, and this further creates some confusion. Let's take a closer look. On one hand, God's Word says:

Do not judge, or you too will be judged. For in the same way you judge others, you will be judged, and with the measure you use, it will be measured to you. Why do you look at the speck of sawdust in your brother's eye and pay no attention to the plank in your own eye? How can you say to your brother, "Let me take the speck out of your eye," when all the time there is a plank in your own eye? You hypocrite, first take the plank out of your own eye, and then you will see clearly to remove the speck from your brother's eye (Matt 7:1-5 NIV).

In this Scripture, God calls us to personal conversion for our sins before judging someone else for a sin we are equally guilty of committing. On the other hand, in Galatians 6:1, we read, "Brothers, if someone is caught in a sin, you who are spiritual should restore him gently." This passage goes on to say, "But watch yourself, or you also may be tempted. Carry each other's burdens, and in this way, you will fulfill the law of Christ. If anyone thinks he is something when he is nothing, he deceives himself" (v. 2-3). This passage speaks of the humility and gentleness necessary in approaching people who have fallen away from the grace of God and also the importance of helping to carry their burdens by supporting and praying for them.

I believe it is in the semantics that we get most caught up in this debate about whether to judge or not to judge. The word judge, according to the Merriam-Webster dictionary, means "to form an estimate or evaluation of; especially to form a negative opinion about."[44] The problem with "judging" others is that it holds a negative connotation that can be misunderstood and inadvertently carried forth in a harsh, condescending, rude, or prideful way. Unfortunately, when that happens, it causes more harm and division than its intended purpose, which is to lovingly help that person restore holiness and unity with God.

Instead of "judging and confronting" the sinner, God calls us to "admonish and help" the sinner toward conversion. Do you notice the difference? Perhaps they are essentially the same thing, but the key is in the language and approach that we use. It is critically important to use words and tone of voice that project a loving, compassionate, and respectful message to the recipient.

What does it take to be true to one's convictions and beliefs and yet approach a person with compassion and acceptance? We can first listen with empathy and understanding. Ask questions. Be supportive. God calls us to "Be completely humble and gentle; be patient, bearing with one another in love. Make every effort to keep the unity of the Spirit through the bond of peace" (Eph 4:2-3). God wants us to live at peace with all of our brothers and sisters, in our families, community, and the whole world. It is not an easy task by any means, but it is a calling we can continually strive to achieve. While God calls us to speak in truth, He also desires for us to see the beauty and goodness of God in each person we encounter.

If there is a situation where one feels God's calling to admonish someone, it must be done with truth, yet compassion and empathy, not harshness or rudeness. The person must be approached with a heart of humility, grace, and love. Make sure the focus isn't on disappointment in the person, inadvertently elevating oneself to a more righteous position. Having social graces and communication skills, as well as being "gentle and humble in heart" (Matt 11:29) like Jesus, is essential for the message to be communicated in an effective manner that produces positive results. The relationship and trust between these two people are factors that contribute to the open reception of the message. It may be best to consult with someone in a religious leadership position and pray about it, seeking the appropriate time and place to have the conversation and not let it happen in a knee-jerk reactionary manner.

An article published by the Roman Catholic Diocese of Portland called "Admonish the Sinner" is excellent, brief, and provides a few practical tips. It reads, "Admonishing the sinner is not to judge but to be supportive in helping others find their way and correct their mistakes." A quote by Bishop Robert Deeley, in this same article, speaks of the importance of having the right motives and disposition of the heart. He says,

> Remember that the goal is not to tell others how poorly they are acting. Neither is the goal to feel superior. Rather, the goal is to win the sinner back from a destructive path and remind them of the forgiveness of sins that is available to all who repent. The goal is salvation. As such, to admonish sinners is to call lovingly to those in danger and draw them back from the edge of an abyss.[45]

In summary, there is great merit in having the proper disposition to love and help our brothers and sisters find their way to the goodness of our merciful and forgiving Father. Holy Scripture tells us to "remember this: Whoever turns a sinner from the error of their way will save them from death and cover over a multitude of sins" (James 5:20). Wow, that's a tall order! God gives us each other to help one another in this journey of life. It's important for each of us to check our motives and be gentle, loving, and compassionate so that our message is received with an open mind and heart and brings people closer to the heart of Jesus and not further away.

Putting It into Practice:

If someone feels God is calling them to admonish a sinner, they can approach this person by saying, "I love you and I want the best for you. I feel _____ (i.e., concerned) about/when _____ (address the behavior- lie, steal, cheat, drunkenness- not the person), and I want you to experience all life has to offer by being close to God's heart and His will for your life. Please pray about _____ (describe the sin). Here is what God's Word says about it _____ (reference Scripture). I pray that God will be with you, helping you through this situation, and guiding you to His will for your life. I love you. Thank you for listening to me."

PRAYER: "Dear Lord. Help us to live with tolerance and acceptance for one another. Help us to remember that we're all humans on this journey together, no one person is better than another. Keep our motives pure and holy, seeking to share your love and goodness in all we do. Amen."

VERSE: "Instead, speaking the truth in love, we will grow to become in every respect the mature body of him who is the head, that is, Christ. From Him, the whole body joined and held together by every supporting ligament, grows and builds itself up in love, as each part does its work" (Eph 4:15-16).

Love God First

"You shall have no other gods before me" (Exodus 20:3).

First and foremost, it's essential for us to focus on God, not ourselves or others. As we strive to do His will and please Him above all else and all others, we experience His goodness, grace, and peace. Scripture states, "Love the Lord your God with all your heart and with all your soul and with all your strength and with all your mind;" (Luke 10:27).

Loving God with all of our *heart* means having a sincere desire and compassion to truly know and love Him in a deep and personal way.

Loving God with all of our *soul* means that in the deepest recesses of our being, we desire to please God and give Him all of ourselves.

Loving God with all of our *strength* means that we are not weary but that we persevere in the fight for "what is true…honorable…right… pure…lovely, and admirable" (Phil 4:8 NLT). We strive to stay in love with God and continue our spiritual growth toward holiness each day of our lives.

Loving God with all of our *mind* means that we fight back fear, doubt, and lies of the enemy. We persevere in mental toughness to know and understand who our loving God is and what He desires for our lives.

God knows how distractible we can be as human beings. We are pulled back and forth like the wind. Unless we have one guiding source for spiritual direction, life will be even more haphazard and confusing than it already is. When we seek God first, everything else falls into place. Then, we have one source for guidance in our thoughts, priorities, attitudes, and actions. If we put ourselves above God, then we fall into pride and self-seeking behaviors. If we put others before God, then we are people-pleasing and live to serve people rather than our loving, wise, and compassionate, Almighty Father. God will show us the way when we put Him first. "I will instruct you and teach you in the way you should go; I will counsel you with my loving eye on you" (Psalm 32:8 NIV). Everything else makes sense when we put God first.

When we continue to seek God and make Him our best friend, we feel His presence more and more. We can grow closer to Christ through prayer, meditation, reflection, attending Mass, receiving the sacraments, and studying the Bible. We can read reputable books, or participate in worship through Eucharistic Adoration or Christian songs. We can also nurture our spiritual growth and connections with other Godly people through faith formation groups. These practices can not only exponentially deepen our faith and love of God but also bring us peace, hope, and joy in the process. This is what God desires for our lives.

Love Others Unconditionally

"All of you, be like-minded, be sympathetic, love one another, be compassionate and humble" (1 Peter 3:8).

Do you remember the song "They'll know we are Christians by our love?"[46] What would happen if Christians everywhere embraced and lived out this identity? What a wonderful world it would be! Love necessitates that we are caring and kind, understanding and patient. First Corinthians 13:4-8 describes love so beautifully:

> Love is patient, love is kind. It does not envy, it does not boast, it is not proud. It does not dishonor others, it is not self-seeking, it is not easily angered, it keeps no record of wrongs. Love does not delight in evil but rejoices with the truth. It always protects, always trusts, always hopes, always perseveres. Love never fails.

Love others unconditionally. This is especially challenging if someone is irritable or rude. As hard as it is, God calls us to love those who are most difficult to love. We don't know the hardships someone is experiencing. Look at their strengths and what is good about them. God is in everyone and he loves everyone. "But to you who are listening I say: Love your enemies, do good to those who hate you, bless those who curse you, pray for those who mistreat you" (Luke 6:27-28). I believe this is one of the most challenging callings as a Christian. We likely all struggle with this. Persevere and ask God's help. He will help us.

Love is shown in both our words and our actions. Love is reflected in the verbal and non-verbal messages we send. Love and respect are reflected in our tone of voice, facial expressions, and physical gestures.

Are we reflecting love in all we do? Do we have pure motives and desire what's best for others? Do we have their best intentions at heart, even when it is a difficult conversation? That's a good thing to reflect upon. God says, "Dear children, let's not merely say that we love each other; let us show the truth by our actions" (1 John 3:18 NLT). The highest good is willing the good of others and helping them to see the goodness of God. Let me clarify that this may require us to be firm and assertive, but this shouldn't ever require us to be harsh or rude. Love, at its best, requires that we speak the truth and wills the best of the other person, and that is sometimes something people do not want to hear.

God calls us to demonstrate a love that involves listening and understanding others rather than to formulate a response. Putting others' needs before our own, as Jesus did, is the greatest gift we can give to others. By listening with the character quality of attentiveness, we show that we value that person and what they have to say is important. We are putting their needs before our own.

"Spouting off before listening to the facts is both shameful and foolish" (Prov 18:13). Do we listen to others with an open heart? Do we show openness, compassion, and kindness to others even if they have different lifestyles or viewpoints? What if they have different political or religious beliefs than us? It's not easy to always show love in these situations.

When it comes to disagreements about matters of religion, it can be helpful to share our hearts with people to tell them why an aspect of our faith is so important to us and not be defensive or try to convince them to think like us. Rather, share from the heart and respect their viewpoint. Be inquisitive and ask questions about their beliefs and faith journey. Be curious, be interested, and have a caring heart.

God's Word says that He will know we are His disciples by the manner in which we love one another. How much do we strive to love like Jesus?

PRAYER: Lord Jesus, help us to love others unconditionally as you do. When it is most difficult, send the Holy Spirit to be at our side, guiding, guarding, and protecting us. Amen."

VERSE: "A new command I give you: Love one another. As I have loved you, so you must love one another. By this everyone will know that you are my disciples, if you love one another" (John 13:34-35 NIV).

Don't Forget to Love Yourself

"God created man in his own image, in the image of God He created him" (Gen 1:27 KJV).

God is our Father, and we are His beloved children. We are made in His image and likeness. God is loving, forgiving, and merciful to us, so it stands to reason that He also desires us to be loving, forgiving, and merciful to ourselves.

When we love God as our heavenly Father, we consequently love ourselves in a whole new way as His beloved children. God wants us to love ourselves because He knows it is the best way to live in harmony with ourselves and others. Self-love also improves our well-being. An article by VCU Health states that "there is a substantial body of psychological research that shows self-compassion and self-love do have a strong impact on our mental health and our emotional state, both in terms of decreasing anxiety, depression, anger and loneliness and also increasing support and encouragement for ourselves."[47]

Holding onto guilt is the opposite of self-love and it affects our self-esteem. When we feel inferior or insecure, we often compare ourselves to others. Throw away the measuring stick and stop comparing. You are a beloved child of God with special gifts, skills, and abilities, and a heart, soul, and mind that make you unique and wonderful. Coveting what others have is a trap for discontentment, but nurturing and valuing the gifts God has given us brings contentment and peace.

Did you know that God loves us no matter what? "Nothing in all creation will ever be able to separate us from the love of God that is revealed in Christ Jesus our Lord" (Rom 8:39 NLT). What a beautiful promise of God.

PRAYER: "Lord God, we know that your greatest commandment is to love. Help us to strive to love without the judgment that drives people further from your love and your Church. Help us to love others unconditionally with acceptance, tolerance, and compassion. May we remember to love you first and that your great love will then flow through us to others like a ray of sunshine, warming their hearts and filling us back up with the joy of the Lord. Amen."

VERSE: "And over all these virtues put on love, which binds them all together in perfect unity" (Col 3:14 NIV).

6

Making a Positive Difference

"In the same way, let your light shine before others, that they may see your good deeds and glorify your Father in heaven" (Matt 5:16).

We are the "Face" and "Voice" of the Church

From the beginning of time, people's perceptions of a business, organization, or educational establishment are primarily defined by the most visible representatives of that entity. Think about when we walk into a Walmart and see the greeter. That greeter at that moment is the face of Walmart. We have an immediate impression and feeling about the store from the moment we walk in. The same holds true for a front desk secretary at a school. This person is the first person we will likely meet and interact with when we walk into that school. In both of these examples, our first impression is determined by the first person we interact with. That said, in the example of the school, everyone else, such as the teaching staff, administrators, school board, custodians, and coaches, all set the tone and feeling within that environment. It's no different in any other school, business, or organization. Its employees, members, and affiliates all represent that establishment. Churches are no different. In the Catholic Church, the pope, cardinals, bishops, priests, religious lay persons, and especially those most visible to the community play a role in defining the public's (and an individual's) perception of Catholicism. But beyond that, each person who identifies as Catholic also defines the faith. The things we say and the way we act all impact others' perceptions of the faith, for better or worse.

Both religious and secular laity have a responsibility to be a good exemplar of faith to others. This goes beyond Catholicism to all Christians. We are the body of Christ, the living church here on this earth. We are called to represent the Church in a loving, positive light. We are the Church's "face and voice." God calls us to be messengers and ambassadors for Christ with each of our actions. We are to be a light in the darkness.

The messages we send and the language we use are critical. God's Word says, "May these words of my mouth and this meditation of my heart be pleasing in your sight, Lord, my Rock and my Redeemer" (Ps 19:14).

Our words can build up or tear down. Having worked extensively in character development within the schools, I would often see elementary teachers using a book called "How Full is Your Bucket?"[48] The basic premise is that all interactions with others matter. It's important to consider whether or not our interactions are filling up or withdrawing from other people's well-being "buckets."

Catholics and Christians have a history of being perceived as intolerant and unaccepting of particular groups of people. Even within the Church, there is division. Sadly, some churches are still segregated by the ethnicity of their parishioners. We must rewrite this story, and it starts with our actions. All Catholics and Christians represent the Church of Christ, not just the priests and those in leadership roles. Let us strive to be peacemakers, reflecting God's light in our actions and fostering unity and love as disciples of Christ.

As Christians, it's essential to be continually building FAITH, HOPE, and LOVE in our homes, workplaces, and community. To discern this, we can ask ourselves these questions: As a Christian, how do we make others feel when they are around us? How are we influencing their faith? Are we positively influencing and supporting their faith? Do they feel the love of Jesus by being in our presence? Do we bring God's message of hope into their hearts? Are we a good example of Christianity in this world? Strive to reflect God's love and grace. It's not only what we say but how we say it in our nonverbal messages as well. Our tone, inflection, and facial expressions all add to the received message.

A new friend of mine, whom I met through writing this book, shared with me a story of when her boyfriend of 11 years was on his deathbed. She, along with his family and friends, were at his hospital bedside when they asked her, "Are you Catholic?" When she said "no," they dismissed her with an "I'm not surprised" expression, and an awkward silence followed. She will never forget the way she was treated, and it was the non-verbal messages that hurt her more than the question they asked. She shared with me how she felt rejected and alone, inferior, ostracized, and not included as "one of them."

I've heard of other instances where people have called church rectories only to be met with an unkind, abrupt voice on the other end of the phone. One such example involved a young woman who called her very own parish to get married there, and the woman she talked with was so unkind that she decided to get married somewhere else! We need to remember that every message we send to others has the power to lift up or tear down, to welcome or turn off, to accept or reject. "Let no corrupting talk come out of your mouths, but only such as is good for building up, as fits the occasion, that it may give grace to those who hear" (Eph 4:29).

Maya Angelou is commonly attributed to saying, "I've learned that people will forget what you said, people will forget what you did, but people will never forget how you made them feel." The communication we deliver with our verbal and nonverbal messages could be received in a completely different manner than we intend it to be understood. Our facial expressions, tone of voice, and the inflection in our words often say more than our words themselves. What truly matters is how others perceive the message we send because, in reality, it's the only message they hear and the only one that matters.

In holy Scripture, we are reminded of God's Words, "But I tell you that everyone will have to give account on the day of judgment for every empty word they have spoken" (Matt 12:36). "Therefore encourage one another and build each other up, just as in fact you are doing" (1 Thess 5:11).

Are we representing the Church in a way that pleases God? Do we see God in everyone? Do we treat people as if God is in them? Do we represent the Catholic Church and Christianity in a manner that draws others in or repels them? Are we striving to be loving and accepting of all God's children, or do we act better than others with overly self-righteous, critical, or harsh words and actions?

"If you claim to be religious but don't control your tongue, you are fooling yourself, and your religion is worthless. Pure and genuine religion in the sight of God the Father means caring for orphans and widows in their distress and refusing to let the world corrupt you" (James 1:26-27 NLT).

As a people, we need to move from division to unity and harshness to love and respect. Let us be stewards of peace and unity, first in our hearts, then in our families, and in our community, which spreads to the world. When I was president of the Character Council of Western New York, we created a tagline that reads "Better ME, Better WE, Better

COMMUNITY."[49] It starts with each of us. Like a chain reaction of kindness, it just takes one person and one spark to ignite the flame of love, unity, and peace in the world. Let us start today by being a part of that positive change in the world, and may we move forward with greater discernment and intentions to love as Jesus loved.

PRAYER: "Lord Jesus, your word reminds us how powerful our communication is. Help us control our tongue and give us the grace to think before we speak. Grant us wisdom and right judgment, making sure that what we say is true, necessary, kind, and helpful. May we represent Catholicism and Christianity in an admirable manner that builds your kingdom here on earth. Amen."

VERSE: "Death and life are in the power of the tongue," (Prov 18:21 NKJV).

Focus on What is Within Our Control

It's important to focus on what is within our control and the positive influence we can have in other's lives. Let go of things that are out of our control and pray about them instead. Try not to "fix" others. That's God's role. We need to work on self-improvement first and lead by example, being careful not to act self-righteous. Many Catholic and Christian songs and prayers remind us of the importance of being that instrument of peace, love, pardon, faith, hope, and joy to others.

Be cautious about looking at others and what they're doing, which can lead to judgment and comparison. Yes, we do want to help others in their faith journey, but we have to get ourselves right first. God has given each of us a unique personality and strengths to live a life that is uniquely our own. He wants us to blossom and grow spiritually, emotionally, intellectually, and physically to be our best selves and live our best lives.

The gifts He has given us will also help us to lead by example and make a positive difference in this world. I can personally attest that when I am operating within my areas of strength, I have more energy and enthusiasm for my work. I am energized and not drained from daily tasks. I feel good that I am making a positive difference, and I experience more peace and joy daily.

If you are interested to know what your unique strengths are, a free assessment can be found at https://high5test.com/.[50]

Understand and Operate Within Our Spiritual Gifts

"Each of you should use whatever gift you have received to serve others, as faithful stewards of God's grace in its various forms" (1 Peter 4:10 NIV).

It's important to know how God is calling us to be disciples. A great way to find this out is to do a spiritual gifts test such as https://spiritualgifts test.com/.[51] Once we understand and operate within our spiritual gifts, we will bloom and grow as the person God created us to be. Joy and fulfillment are the beautiful outcomes of working and serving others through our spiritual gifts.

God wants us to shine our light for all to see. Matthew 5:14 and 5:16 read, "You are the light of the world. A town built on a hill cannot be hidden...In the same way, let your light shine before others, that they may see your good deeds and glorify your Father in heaven."

Strive to be confident in the gifts our Lord has given you. Please do not be shy and hide them for fear that others may feel inferior. Shining our light by operating within our gifts will also inspire others to rise up and seek the joy and fulfillment that we are experiencing in our lives.

Develop Knowledge and Understanding of Faith

"The heart of the discerning acquires knowledge, for the ears of the wise seek it out" (Prov 18:15).

Developing knowledge, understanding God, and growing in our faith and spirituality requires that we take initiative. It's not something that we can be passive about, waiting and hoping something will happen. Just as seeds need water and sunshine to grow and bloom, so too our spiritual self needs nourishment to develop and grow. Without it, our faith will likely wither and die.

By taking the initiative and seeking opportunities in our faith community to learn about Jesus and grow our faith and trust in Him, we have a much better chance of living in the peace and joy of Christ. Strive to be a life-long learner by engaging in faith formation opportunities offered through your parish, faith community, or even online resources. My favorite faith formation activities have been *Christ Renews His Parish Welcome* retreat, Eucharistic Adoration, faith sharing groups, morning Mass, Mission, Bible app devotionals, and teaching Confirmation classes. Through each of these experiences, I have grown in my personal relationship with and love for Jesus. I have made lifelong friends with whom I communicate nearly every week, and my prayer life has grown exponentially. My faith is no longer a burden, chore, or task to be checked off the list. It is the greatest blessing and joy!

PRAYER: "Lord, give us the courage and energy to seek out and participate in faith formation activities that will increase our faith and love for you. Help us to build your kingdom here on earth and be an instrument of your peace. May we grow in goodness, and may the fruit of the Holy Spirit be evidence of your presence and work in our lives. Amen."

VERSE: "For the LORD gives wisdom; from his mouth come knowledge and understanding" (Prov 2:6 NKJV).

7

Mindset Reset

"Finally, brothers and sisters, whatever is true, whatever is noble, whatever is right, whatever is pure, whatever is lovely, whatever is admirable—if anything is excellent or praiseworthy—think about such things" (Phil 4:8 NIV).

Mindset is Powerful

The mind is incredibly powerful. It is so powerful that what we choose to focus our thoughts on influences every aspect of our lives. Our thoughts influence our feelings, decisions, and actions. They are all connected.

I'd like to tell a story of a personal mental crisis I experienced after leaving my full-time tenured school counseling position. It was a job that I loved in so many ways. I especially appreciated getting to know my students personally and helping them through the challenges of middle school. The following fall, after I resigned from my position, I found myself in a tailspin mentally and emotionally.

It was the first few months of a new school year when all the other teachers and support staff went back to their jobs, and I started my new business as a Stress Management Coach. It was an exciting time but a terrifying and challenging time as well. It was a time of incredible vulnerability and uncertainty regarding what the future would hold, and I was all alone in this private practice venture.

As the days and weeks progressed, I noticed something happening mentally and physically. Ironically, even though I was a stress management coach, I started having what felt like panic attacks immediately upon waking. Thoughts would flood my head about what I had done. Thoughts like, "Are you crazy?" "You left a full-time tenured job in a school!" "How are you going to pay your bills?" "How are you going to get enough clients to keep things going?"

Each day, things got progressively worse, and the worried self-talk continued to escalate to the point where I was getting chest pains. It all came to a head one day when I realized that I needed to take action. I needed to practice what I was preaching, do my breathing techniques, and change my mindset. I certainly didn't want to end up in the hospital again with cardiac symptoms like I did ten years prior.

Once I recognized what was happening and that the way I was feeling, including the physical symptoms, were all starting with my thoughts, I was able to take back control. I changed my thinking and self-talk to "You got this!" "You are intelligent, capable, qualified, caring and have what it takes to be successful at this." "Get up and start your day." "Make it a great day."

I was reminded of the *Words of Wisdom* we would read in school over the morning announcements. We would say, "Make it a great day or not. The choice is yours."[52] I kept thinking of that over and over. What great advice! I put that advice into action. I put my trust in God and started praying more and putting my thoughts and decisions into His hands. My favorite three promises of God that got me through that rough time are:

- "Trust in the LORD with all your heart and lean not on your own understanding; in all your ways submit to him, and he will make your paths straight" (Prov 3:5-6 NKJV).
- "Do not be anxious about anything, but in every situation, by prayer and petition, with thanksgiving, present your requests to God. And the peace of God, which transcends all understanding, will guard your hearts and your minds in Christ Jesus" (Phil 4:6-7 NIV).
- "Be still, and know that I am God;" (Ps 46:1).

There have been multiple situations in my lifetime where God came to my rescue and helped me change my mindset. In turn, my life was positively influenced. This is partially because every success we have increases our self-esteem and self-efficacy. We gain wisdom along the journey of life. Learning from each life experience helps us to be even better and more resilient. Knowing we have control of our thoughts, and that by changing them we can positively influence our lives at any moment, is incredibly empowering.

Think about the power of thoughts in your life. Are you the type of person who looks at the glass half full or half empty? Think about one area of your life where your thoughts are in control and the result takes you down a path to feelings and actions you'd like to change. Are there any thoughts about your faith life and spirituality that don't serve you well? Remember, our thoughts, feelings, and behaviors are all connected. We can intercept this process at any point by changing our thinking.

PRAYER: "Lord, help us to realize the power of our mindset and the connection to our heart. Empower us with positive and confident thoughts that honor you."

VERSE: "May these words of my mouth and this meditation of my heart be pleasing in your sight, Lord, my Rock and my Redeemer" (Ps 19:14).

Taking Control of Our Thoughts

As we continue this journey of life, taking control of our thoughts will impact every area of our lives. Improving our thought life can benefit us physically, emotionally, mentally, and spiritually, affecting our whole well-being! Life is a journey and every moment is an opportunity for positive action and change. It's no different with our thoughts. Research shows that one's mindset plays a significant role in determining that person's life outcome. "By understanding, adapting, and shifting your mindset, you can improve your health, decrease your stress, and become more resilient to life's challenges."[53]

The other great news is that our thoughts are not facts. So often, we dwell on an anxious thought so long that we actually believe it to be true or think that it will happen. This couldn't be further from the truth. In fact, studies show that the majority of what we worry about never happens, and when our worries do come true, the outcome and how we handle it is usually better than expected.[54]

Our perception of a situation is formed based on how we perceive, process, and think about an experience, a conversation, or an event. It is our interpretation of the situation. Sometimes, our perceptions are spot on, but often, they are not accurate at all. Numerous times, my coaching clients realized that their worried thoughts and perceptions were not serving them well and were simply untrue. One example is when we perceive someone to be mad at us, resulting in a strained relationship, only to find out it was just a misperception on our part.

Many factors contribute to our perception of a situation. Often, the message received is very different from the message the sender intended to be heard. Take control of your thoughts, gain wisdom and understanding, and communicate concerns to other people to verify their feelings before jumping to a conclusion. The bottom line is that most of the fears we have are not true, and many of the things we worry about will never happen. We have to protect our minds and ask the Holy Spirit to help us have the mindset of Christ. Having the mindset of Christ looks like Philippians 4:6–7: "Have no anxiety at all, but in everything, with prayer and petition, with thanksgiving, make your requests known to God. Then the peace of Christ that surpasses all understanding will guard your hearts and minds in Christ Jesus."

During Mass, and after the Lord's Prayer, the presiding priest prays a "Prayer for Peace" over the congregation saying, "Deliver us Lord, we pray, from every evil, graciously grant peace in our days, that, by the help of your mercy, we may be always free from sin and safe from all distress, as we await the blessed hope and the coming of our Savior, Jesus Christ."[55] What a beautiful prayer on behalf of the entire assembly of people, invoking God's mercy and peace for all present. This prayer touches my heart in a special way and gives me peace and comfort every time I hear it.

Having the mindset of Christ not only helps us rightly interpret a situation, but it also helps us make the right decisions…holy and good and righteous decisions. This will likely be a daily challenge for all of us, due to our imperfect and fallen nature. However, by invoking God's help and submitting to His will through prayer, God's grace will be at work in our minds and hearts to bring us closer and closer to His Holy, perfect, and pleasing will.

PRAYER: "Lord, help us to take control of our thoughts to be healthy and in line with your will. Continually renew our minds to reflect the mindset of Christ."

VERSE: "Do not conform to the pattern of this world, but be transformed by the renewing of your mind. Then you will be able to test and approve what God's will is—his good, pleasing and perfect will" (Rom 12:2).

Perspective is Key

Our perspective, in contrast to our perception, is our point of view. Our perspective is an overarching belief system that evolves and changes over time. It responds to different influences and information that we are exposed to and experience. Consider this: Is there an area in your spiritual life where you could gather additional information to gain a clearer, more accurate perspective on your faith?

Like our perception of a situation, our perspective also impacts our feelings, beliefs, and attitudes. It influences our decisions and actions and determines the direction of our lives. Everything in life can be viewed from multiple perspectives. The great news is that our perspective can be shifted over time by changing our thoughts about that person, place, or situation.

For example, have we ever glanced at someone who walked into church late? When things like this happen, do we think, "How rude of that person to walk in late?" or "They are interrupting my prayer time," or do we say, "Thank you, Jesus, that she/he made it to Mass this morning." Or, if we encounter someone who has had an abortion, do we think, "This is a sin. How could the mother be so selfish?" or do we say, "I'm sad this woman thought that this was the best alternative and I pray for the soul of the unborn baby and the mother's emotional healing." These subtle shifts change our whole perspective and are likely to bring peace to our minds rather than frustration. The following are additional examples of situations and how we can shift our perspective by making a simple adjustment in our thoughts and self-talk:

Marital Strife:

Hurtful: "Why can't my husband (wife) do anything right?"

Helpful: "Lord, help me to have patience and understanding and to see the good in him (her), and to calmly discuss the areas that trouble me."

Children:

Hurtful: "When are my children going to grow up and move out? I don't know if I can take this anymore."

Helpful: "Lord, help me to have patience and enjoy every moment with my children. Help me to realize that someday, when they move out, I will miss these days and regret that I didn't enjoy them more."

Job/Career:

Hurtful: "I hate this job and can't wait to leave/retire."

Helpful: "Lord, help me to notice the good things about my work and to see my value."

Young Generation of "Nones":[56]

Hurtful: "It's terrible that young people these days believe they don't need any religion."

Helpful: "Lord, help me to show the younger generation the importance of faith. Help them to see my strong faith through the example I live."

Catholic Church:

Hurtful: "The Catholic Church is corrupt."

Helpful: "The Catholic Church is not perfect, but it is filled with many holy, righteous people who can help me build a stronger faith."

As shown in these examples, our thoughts hold immense power in shaping our perspectives, which in turn influence our attitudes, beliefs, and behaviors. Our perspectives are constantly evolving and shaped by our life experiences, role models, and other influences. Each of us is at a unique point in our thoughts, beliefs, and faith journey, and these beliefs naturally change over time based on what we learn, listen to, read, and experience.

Given the ongoing accumulation of life experiences, it's crucial to be mindful of the influences we allow into our lives and whether they align with the direction we want our lives to take. To live a virtuous, holy life, Scripture advises: "Guard your heart above all else, for it determines the course of your life" (Prov 4:23 NLT). Guarding our hearts means being selective about what we allow our eyes to see and our ears to hear, as these are gateways to our hearts. What we consume affects our perspective.

To guard our hearts effectively, it's essential to fill our minds with things that are true, holy, and uplifting. It can be challenging to know the right course of action and how to maintain God's perspective, but the Bible is an invaluable resource, offering guidance and answers to life's questions. Additionally, practicing gratitude is a wonderful virtue and research-based strategy that can significantly improve our outlook on life. It's a simple practice that can shift our perspective and transform our experience and enjoyment of life for the better.

PRAYER: "Lord God, you have given us a beautiful mind to use for your glory. Help us to gain the perspective of Christ so that we may honor you and live with peace and joy on this earth, loving others as you love us."

VERSE: "Let this mind be in you, which was also in Christ Jesus" (Phil 2:5 KJV).

8

A Joy-Full Life

> *"But the advocate, the Holy Spirit, whom the Father will send in my name, will teach you all things and will remind you of everything I have said to you"* (John 14:26 NLT).

The Holy Spirit

Who and what is the Holy Spirit? So many things regarding faith are a mystery, but one thing I sense for sure is when the power of the Holy Spirit is working in and through me. I would have never had the courage to leave a well-paying consulting position to start back on my own as a Christian Life and Mindset Coach had I not felt the prompting of the Holy Spirit to pursue that path.

God calls us to continually seek the guidance of The Holy Spirit and to keep striving to know and love Him: Father, Son, and Holy Spirit. God loves us so much, and He knew this journey of life would be very difficult, so He gave us an advocate and helper to be with us at all times. "And I will ask the Father, and he will give you another Advocate, who will never leave you" (John 14:16).

This helper, the Holy Spirit, is the third person of the Holy Trinity that God gives us so that we will never be alone. The Holy Spirit helps us to grow in the theological virtues of faith, hope, and love. When we pray and earnestly invoke the help of the Holy Spirit, He molds us into the image of Christ. This process never ends and is a continual development throughout our entire lives.

A simple way that I like to imagine the Holy Spirit is that of a good angel on our right shoulder. The Holy Spirit is considered the "spirit of truth" as described in John 16:13, "When the Spirit of truth comes, he will guide you into all truth. He will not speak on his own but will tell you what he has heard. He will tell you about the future."

The Holy Spirit lives in us, but we might not feel His presence. We need to call upon the Holy Spirit to help us in our decision-making, and it is that still small voice in our conscience that guides us to do the right thing and avoid the wrong thing. We can choose to listen to the promptings of the Holy Spirit, or we can certainly choose not to as well. Forces of good and evil exist all around us.

Another way I imagine the Holy Spirit intervening is similar to the forces of good versus evil in animated movies. Opposing forces are present in every one of these movies I've watched. Thankfully, as depicted in these movies and promised through biblical Scripture, God's goodness and power are stronger than any evil in this world. It doesn't mean every person will choose the holy and righteous route. God gives us free will. We are imperfect humans, fallen and tempted every day to follow sinful ways. What makes this even more difficult is that sin is often disguised as something fun and attractive to pursue. This is one of the reasons we need to seek God's will and the guidance of the Holy Spirit so earnestly.

Think about every decision we need to make. Do we walk toward holiness and the light of God's truth and goodness, or turn away and follow our human desires? God tells us the truth when He says, "I am the light of the world. Whoever follows me will never walk in darkness, but will have the light of life" (John 8:12 NIV). I believe the Holy Spirit will guide us to that light through our conscience when we invoke His help and earnestly seek to know, understand, and do what is right in God's eyes. Certainly, it helps a whole lot to understand what God's Word says in the Holy Bible. I believe the Bible holds every instruction for living a good, holy, and virtuous life. Therefore, by combining prayer and invoking the help of the Holy Spirit, along with knowing God's Word, we can strive toward the grace of living a holy and righteous life.

PRAYER: "Thank you, Lord, for the gift of the Holy Spirit who lives within us at all times. Continue to be ever so close to us, guiding, guarding, and keeping us from evil."

VERSE: "(May the Holy Spirit) equip you with everything good for doing his will, and may he work in us what is pleasing to him, through Jesus Christ, to whom be glory for ever and ever! Amen" (Heb 13:21).

Grow in the Fruits of the Holy Spirit

Growing in faith and seeking desires of the spirit rather than the flesh is a lifelong process. When we are close to God and live in harmony with the Holy Spirit, according to His word, we will see the evidence of that in our lives. Some biblical scholars do not feel we can develop these attributes on our own. I agree that we cannot develop these through our own accord. They are a direct result of the Holy Spirit working in our lives. We do, however, need to be open to the prompting of the Holy Spirit and live with an intentional desire to know, love, and please God. We can learn about these virtues and, as an active participant, be receptive to God's grace and the nurturing of these virtues in our lives. These "fruits" are listed in Galatians 5:22-23 and include love, joy, peace, patience, kindness, goodness, gentleness, faithfulness, and self-control. These fruits are the visible signs of the Holy Spirit's presence and work in our lives. As we welcome the Holy Spirit to transform and mold us into His image and likeness, with a sincere desire to be transformed, the holiness that our lives exemplify will be noticed and desired by other people. These fruits of the Holy Spirit give us a beautiful reason to desire oneness with God and experience a fulfilling life of HOPE.

Let us take a closer look at each FRUIT OF THE SPIRIT:

LOVE

Love seeks the highest good for others, no matter their behavior, and gives freely without seeking anything in return. This "agape" love is a choice and is freely given to all, never considering the worth or worthiness of its object or recipient. According to Scripture, "Love is patient, love is kind. It does not envy, it does not boast, it is not proud. It does not dishonor others, it is not self-seeking, it is not easily angered, it keeps no record of wrongs. Love does not delight in evil but rejoices with the truth. It always protects, always trusts, always hopes, always perseveres" (1 Cor 13:4-7).

JOY

True joy is rooted in God and goes deeper than worldly happiness, which is based on our circumstances and emotions. True joy is lasting because it comes from God through trusting in Him and living according to His word and His will. How exciting it is to know that we can experience joy no matter what is happening around us. Scripture says, "Be full of joy in the Lord always. I will say again, be full of joy. Let everyone see that you are gentle and kind. The Lord is coming soon" (Phil 4:4-5).

PEACE

Peace is a state of tranquility and calmness, having a sense of wholeness. When we have God's peace, we are not shaken by our circumstances or the pressures of life. It is having a sense of security, harmony, and safety that God is with us and for us. "You will keep in perfect peace those whose minds are steadfast, because they trust in you" (Isa 26:3). "Peace I leave with you; my peace I give you. I do not give to you as the world gives. Do not let your hearts be troubled and do not be afraid" (John 14:27).

PATIENCE

When we have patience, we are "slow to anger, abounding in love and faithfulness," (Exodus 34:6). Patience is endurance under difficult circumstances, and maintaining hope without giving in to defeat. Patient people exercise restraint and love instead of revenge. God's Word confirms this as Scripture informs us to "Be completely humble and gentle; be patient, bearing with one another in love" (Eph 4:2).

KINDNESS

Kindness is typically described as being caring and compassionate. Kindness involves action, rather than just a thought or intention to be kind. Jesus was a great example of kindness because he cared for the needy, sick, and marginalized. Kindness can be as simple as smiling and saying "hello" to a stranger. Kindness is one of those things that boomerangs back and blesses the giver as much as the receiver! "Those who are kind benefit themselves, but the cruel bring ruin on themselves" (Prov 11:17).

GOODNESS

Goodness, in simplest terms, is acting with Godly character, being holy, pure, and righteous. It is honorable to strive for goodness (holiness, purity, righteousness) in our words and actions. This can only come from God's grace and a sincere desire from within ourselves to cultivate this spiritual fruit in our inner being and character. Cultivating goodness brings joy through the mere action of "being" good, but its intentions ought to be for the benefit of others, not ourselves. "Therefore, as we have opportunity, let us do good to all people, especially to those who belong to the family of believers" (Gal 6:10).

FAITHFULNESS

Faithfulness as a Fruit of the Spirit refers to our commitment, dependability, and steadfast love for Christ. Even though it is not always easy to believe and feel His presence, God asks that we put our faith, trust, and dependence in Him. "And it is impossible to please God without faith. Anyone who wants to come to him must believe that God exists and that he rewards those who sincerely seek him" (Heb 11:6 NLT).

GENTLENESS

To exhibit gentleness, one needs to be even-tempered and balanced. Gentleness is not weakness but rather power and strength under control. Exhibiting gentleness means pardoning injuries, correcting faults, and acting with tenderness. "Be completely humble and gentle; be patient, bearing with one another in love" (Eph 4:2 NIV).

SELF-CONTROL

When we exhibit self-control, we control and direct our thoughts, words, and actions and act in moderation. We control our fleshly desires and short-term gratifications for the long-term good. This results in lasting joy and peace. "No temptation has overtaken you except what is common to mankind. And God is faithful; he will not let you be tempted beyond what you can bear. But when you are tempted, he will also provide a way out so that you can endure it" (1 Cor 10:13).

In conclusion, if we genuinely want to live a fulfilling life, it is imperative that we continually strive to seek the guidance of the Holy Spirit to cultivate these qualities in our lives. This is a lifelong process, and it's natural for each of us to have strengths and areas for growth as we continue to turn our lives and our will over to God. The goal is not perfection but openness, intentionality, and a sincere desire to invite the Holy Spirit to continually develop these qualities within us throughout our lifetime. As we open ourselves to God's grace and the prompting of the Holy Spirit, we will grow closer to God and thrive, not just survive. We will live our most fulfilling, peaceful, and joy-filled lives!

Reflection: Which of the nine fruits of the Holy Spirit do you see God's light shining forth in your life? Which ones do you ask the Holy Spirit's help to cultivate more fully in your life?

PRAYER: "Lord Jesus, you give us all that is good. You know us better than anyone else. Form us and mold us into the person you want us to become. Help us to grow each day in love, joy, peace, patience, kindness, goodness, faithfulness, gentleness, and self-control. Shine your light through us to be a visible sign of your presence in this world."

VERSE: "And the believers were filled with joy and with the Holy Spirit" (Acts 13:52 NLT).

Note: The Catholic Church recognizes three additional fruits of the spirit, namely generosity, modesty, and chastity. While the Bible does not explicitly list these additional three with the first nine fruits of the spirit, Catholic teaching and tradition recognize these three as important outcomes of the Holy Spirit at work in our lives.

9

Faithfully Healthy

"By faith in the name of Jesus, this man whom you see and know was made strong. It is Jesus' name and the faith that comes through him that has completely healed him, as you can all see" (Acts 3:16 NIV).

Research on the Benefits of Faith

Perhaps you left the Catholic Church long ago and are questioning your next steps in your faith journey. Maybe you are on the verge of jumping ship from your parish or faith community. Perhaps you stopped attending Mass, and you're not quite sure if you want to start attending again at all. Maybe you still practice the faith, but your frustration with the Church has left you disillusioned and lost, wondering if you should continue to participate. Perhaps you've never practiced the Catholic faith at all. No matter where you are in your faith walk, the following are some convincing reasons to hang on to your faith and benefit from better health, too.

It's important to not only consider the benefits of having faith and belonging to a faith community but also to consider the negative impacts on our health and well-being if we don't. There is a body of research showing the benefits of religious involvement and spirituality. Researchers at the Mayo Clinic concluded, "Most studies have shown that religious involvement and spirituality are associated with better health outcomes. This includes greater longevity, better coping skills, and health-related quality of life (even during a terminal illness), less anxiety, depression, and thoughts of suicide."[57]

"In relation to physical health, the majority of studies have found that spirituality/religiousness is related to lower levels of hospitalization and pain, greater survival, and better functional status and cardiovascular outcomes."[58]

Large-scale studies have consistently shown a strong association between being religious and good health. For example, in 2001, Mayo Clinic researchers found that people who regularly attend religious services tend to have lower death rates and hospital admissions, as well as better cardiovascular function and health. They furthermore found that the "increase in death rates among people who never attend religious services compared with those who attend several times a week is comparable to that associated with smoking a pack of cigarettes a day."[59] Wow!

The Catholic Church offers many options for attending religious services, and most parishes have daily Masses. Since attending religious services positively impacts cardiovascular function and reduces hospitalizations and death rates, it is a fair assertion that the Catholic Church also provides opportunities that support health and longevity.

"Religious involvement with God is better for your body in terms of immune functions and reducing loneliness." These positive physical and social/emotional health benefits are reported in a Stanford Report article titled "Deep Faith Beneficial to Health."[60]

I can attest that my spirituality and practice of the faith as a Catholic Christian dramatically reduce my stress and improve my hopefulness and well-being. Through my relationship with God, the support of a community of believers and faith-filled friends, involvement in church ministries, striving to let the Word of God be my guiding light, praying, attending Mass, and participating in the sacraments, I have been able to live a happier and healthier life with more peace, contentment, and joy than I could ever experience on my own without God in my life.

PRAYER: "Lord Jesus, while good health is not the primary reason for practicing our faith, thank you for this added blessing that can help us live a longer life of health and happiness."

VERSE: "This will bring health to your body and nourishment to your bones" (Prov 3:8).

Heaven & Salvation

"I write these things to you who believe in the name of the Son of God so that you may know that you have eternal life" (1 John 5:13).

I know we can't be sure of things with 100% certainty. One might question, "Is there really a heaven?" I guess that's what faith is all about. It's believing in what we can't see or be entirely sure about. Faith is something we have a deep conviction about. When we have faith, we have enough hope in something that we not only accept and believe it in our hearts but also live a life consistent with that belief. It is a beautiful life in my opinion. It's a life of optimism and hope.

Having faith helps us to continue to want to be our best self...not only for ourselves, or for others, but for God. The more we develop

Christ-like qualities, the more loving, patient, and kind we become. It is a synergistic relationship. As we grow in our love for God, we simultaneously grow in love for one another and ourselves, too! This helps not only our spiritual growth but our social/emotional health as well!

Let's talk about heaven and hell for a moment. Whether or not heaven and hell exist, and I believe they do as promised in Scripture, isn't it better to live a life striving to be our best self, loving God and others, seeking to get to heaven, and avoiding hell, in case they do exist? Isn't it better to live a life driven by the desire to please God and live life cultivating virtues such as love, kindness, patience, generosity, righteousness, self-control, gratitude, and compassion?

The lives of millions of people around the world are better because they strive toward holiness, pleasing God, and developing Godly virtues in their lives. For example, we all know that it is better for our health and well-being to have self-control than to be out of control in our eating, drinking, and other fleshly desires. As God saves us from our self-destructive ways, a better life is lived in every way. It is a life of better relationships, more love, more purpose and meaning, better health, more peace and joy, and a fulfillment that could not be imagined without submitting our lives to God. Research also shows that developing other virtues, such as generosity, impacts our health and well-being in several positive ways. Generosity alone boosts mood, self-esteem, and our immune system and reduces stress, anxiety, and blood pressure. Some people experience fewer aches and pains and better sleep too![61]

Will that energy ever be wasted? I don't think so. And, what are the risks if we do believe in heaven and it does not exist? I can't think of any. Can you?

What if hell does, in fact, exist? I know I don't want to live in the eternal fires of damnation, do you? I will do everything I can to live a life that is pleasing to God, surrendering to His will and His way, and eliminating things in my life that drive a wedge between me and God. "If your hand causes you to sin, cut it off. It's better to enter eternal life with only one hand than to go into the unquenchable fires of hell with two hands" (Mark 9:43 NLT). Don't worry, though. I won't cut my hand off.

Belief in heaven also provides positive benefits for us by infusing a hopefulness that we will one day see our deceased loved ones again. Catholic teaching on heaven suggests that this is true. In the Rites of Christian Burial, there is a reference to awaiting the day we are reunited with our deceased loved ones in Jesus Christ. This prayer states: "May we comfort one another with our faith, until we all meet in Christ and are with you and (deceased person's name) forever. Through Christ our Lord."[62]

Since I was a little girl, and especially since my biological father passed away when I was just five years old, I have believed with all my heart that I will see him and my faithfully departed loved ones again. I would have rather lived a life believing this than thinking that I would never see them again. That brings me comfort and so much anticipation and hope. I really feel that I have nothing to lose by believing this, even if, by chance, there isn't a heaven. According to Christian teaching and Scripture though, there indeed is a heaven and hell.

There are several references to the existence of heaven in the Holy Bible. "Jesus told her, 'I am the resurrection and the life. Anyone who believes in me will live, even after dying. Everyone who lives in me and believes in me will never ever die'" (John 11:25-26 NLT). In addition to this promise, Scripture also provides us with instructions on how we get to heaven. In John 14:6, Jesus gives us a clear path to heaven, saying, "I am the way and the truth and the life. No one comes to the Father except through me." This is about so much more than just being a good person, as I often hear people say about the requirements for getting to heaven. Jesus is the only way to God the Father in heaven and we need to believe in Him as our Lord and Savior. We must give up our self-destructive, selfish ways and commit our lives to Him.

We also have the promise of salvation in John 3:16, which reads, "For God so loved the world that he gave his one and only Son, that whoever believes in him shall not perish but have eternal life" (NIV). Here, we have the importance, again, of "believing in Him."

"Let not your hearts be troubled. Believe in God; believe also in me. In my Father's house are many rooms. If it were not so, would I have told you that I go to prepare a place for you? And if I go and prepare a place for you, I will come again and will take you to myself, that where I am you may be also" (John 14:1-3 KJV). Yet again, we have another reference to believing in God and Jesus. We hear that there is a place being prepared for us in the Father's house. It's not just an ordinary place but a magnificent place for those who love and put their hope and trust in God. "No eye has seen, no ear has heard, and no mind has imagined what God has prepared for those who love him" (1 Cor 2:9 NLT).

Believing that there is more at the end of our life on earth is the greatest gift from God we could ever imagine. We all know our life has a limit. It is certain that one day, we will pass away. What do we believe will happen after that? I meet people who are so worried about death. They worry about the pain and suffering, the trauma to family members, and the uncertainty of the afterlife. What a true gift it is to believe in Jesus as our Savior and know that our salvation and life everlasting is with Him in heaven. This promise is the greatest gift we could ever receive. Knowing this creates peace in my heart. It is a peace that surpasses all understanding. "And the peace of God, which surpasses all understanding, will guard your hearts and your minds in Christ Jesus" (Phil 4:7 NKJV).

So, not only is having faith good for our well-being, but it's essential for our salvation, too! I can't imagine living life without this hope and promise from God. I no longer worry about dying. It's so freeing and the greatest gift we could ever hope for.

PRAYER: " *Lord God, you are the source of our hope and salvation. Thank you for the great gift of faith that helps us to live a life of anticipation where we will one day be reunited with you and our faithfully departed loved ones in our eternal home in heaven."*

VERSE: *"There will be no more death, or mourning or crying or pain, for the old order of things has passed away" (Rev 21:4 NIV).*

10

New Beginnings

"Again Jesus spoke to them, saying, "I am the light of the world. Whoever follows me will not walk in darkness, but will have the light of life" (John 8:12).

Positive Change is Always Possible

I genuinely believe that every day, we can start anew. Every day is brimming with possibilities. Possibilities for greater love, greater forgiveness, greater faith, and greater hope. Every day is an opportunity for a new perspective with the beauty of God's light shining through the darkness. We can choose to see it or not. We can choose to look for it or not. We can choose to take off our blinders or not. We can choose to learn more about faith and God's promises in His word, or not.

We have choices with regard to everything we think, do, and say every day. It can be daunting, but it can be gloriously exciting as well. I not only believe that every day is a new opportunity for growth and positive change, but every hour, minute, and moment is as well. When we fall down, do we stay down or do we get back up? When we doubt that God even exists, do we accept that and give up? We have a choice every day. Which choice will we make?

Twelve Solution-Focused Action Items for HOPE, RENEWAL & NEW BEGINNINGS:

1. Seek help to heal the wounds causing anger, resentment, or rejection. Holding on to this pain hurts us more than anyone else.
2. If it is a person or people who have caused you to separate from the Church or your faith, reevaluate the reasons why you left and take steps to forgive and reconcile with those feelings.
3. Open your mind to the beauty of the practices of the Church. Honoring Mary and the saints gives strength to Jesus, not the opposite.
4. Have realistic expectations for yourself in the development of your faith. Taking small daily steps will help. Remember everything worthwhile takes time, so the effort you put in will reap the benefits. God is patient and loving.
5. Resolve feelings of anger, pride, and fear as quickly as possible. These separate us from our best self and our best life living in the grace of God and harmony with others.
6. Love God in His wisdom and teachings first. Then, our love for others and ourselves will follow.
7. Learn to reframe your thoughts to be more positive, hopeful, and optimistic. Focus more on solutions than problems. This one habit can be life-changing.
8. See the best in others, be forgiving, and remember that we are all on this journey together. No one is ever going to think, believe, or behave exactly as we do. Approach everyone with love and

acceptance.

9. Continually strive to be your best self and help others on this journey, too. Grow in the Fruit of the Spirit and strive to live a virtuous life.

10. Take care of yourself. Your body is a temple of the Holy Spirit.

11. Read the Bible (Basic Instruction Before Leaving Earth), and do online or in-person Bible studies to learn about God's Word and promises. The YouVersion Bible App and Hallow App are terrific resources.

12. Grow your faith by attending Mass, becoming part of a worship community, and surround yourself with people who build your Faith, Hope, and Love.

Afterword

If you feel like something is missing from your life, and you've been longing for more fulfillment, joy, and peace, I am confident that the missing piece is a deeper relationship with God. He loves you and wants nothing more than for you to be close to Him...His love, His forgiveness, His compassion, His kindness, His mercy, His hope, and His healing. These are the gifts He gives to us through a relationship with Him.

We cannot find these things in the secular world. Only through faith in God and accepting His Son as our Savior and the Savior of the whole world can we ever truly achieve inner peace, hope, and joy in this life. By inviting the Holy Spirit to be a part of our everyday lives, to abide within us, and helping us each day with our thoughts, words, attitudes, and actions, we can truly live our best life. Life is a journey, not to perfection or even being a "good enough" Catholic or Christian, but to know and love God with all our heart, soul, mind, and strength. In the end, that is all that will really matter.

May the Holy Spirit come to you now, infusing a renewed hope for the life and purpose God has called you to. May you trust in His infinite love and guidance. May you acknowledge your need for His forgiveness for your sins, and His healing mercy and saving grace. May you turn your heart and your life over to Him today and every day for the rest of your life.

I hope and pray that this book has been a blessing to you, and that you will consider sharing it with a loved one. My goal is that this message will reach 10,000 minds and hearts within a year and blossom from there. Will you please share this book with someone you know today?

"I pray that God, the source of hope, will fill you completely with joy and peace because you trust in Him. Then you will overflow with confident hope through the power of the Holy Spirit" (Rom 15:13 NLT). Amen.

With love & gratitude,

Suzanne

Notes

A "GOOD CATHOLIC"

1   M. Boland, "How to Stop Feeling Guilty: 10 Tips," *Healthline* (2022, September 30), https://www.healthline.com/health/mental-health/how-to-stop-feeling-guilty (accessed May 2, 2024).

2   J. J. Boucher, "Grappling with guilt," *Catholic Digest* (2020, October 29), https://ww w.catholicdigest.com/faith/grappling-with-guilt/ (accessed July 8, 2024).

3   John Henry Newman, *An Essay on the Development of Christian Doctrine* (London: James Toovey, 1845), 40.

4   "The Church and the Papacy," *Catholics Come Home*, https://www.catholicscomeho me.org/your-questions/church-teachings/the-church-and-the-papacy/ (accessed August 26, 2024).

A BROKEN CHURCH & HEART

5   "Priest shortage, declining Mass attendance causes Diocese of Buffalo to create plan to merge parishes," *The Dialog* (2024, May 31), https://thedialog.org/national-news /priest-shortage-and-declining-in-mass-attendance-causes-diocese-of-buffalo-to-create-plan-to-merge-parishes/ (accessed July 12, 2024).

6   B. Kettler, "Bankruptcy Protection in the Abuse Crisis: Documents and Articles," *Bishop Accountability*, https://www.bishop-accountability.org/bankruptcy.htm (accessed July 12, 2024).

7   ibid.

8   "We have to root everything in prayer," *The Catholic Sun* (2023, August 10), https://th ecatholicsun.com/we-have-to-root-everything-in-prayer/ (accessed July 12, 2024).

9   "Reformation and Wars of Religion," *Sutori*, https://www.sutori.com/en/story/re formation-wars-of-religion—GzLVCxZihWKrJekBkRoBcTfT (accessed July 11, 2024)

10 ibid.

11 Seven Sisters Apostolate, https://sevensistersapostolate.org/ (accessed August 26, 2024).

12 *Ecclesia semper reformanda est.*, *Wikipedia*, https://en.wikipedia.org/wiki/Ecclesia_s emper_reformanda_est (accessed July 9, 2024)

13 Bishop R. Walter Nickless, "The Church is Always in Need of Renewal- Ecclesia Semper Reformanda," *Catholic Culture* (2009, October 15), https://www.catholiccul ture.org/culture/library/view.cfm?recnum=9162 (accessed July 8, 2024).

14 Pope Francis, *A Gift of Joy and Hope* (2022), Worthy Publishing, p.8.

HEALING AND MOVING FORWARD

15 "Anger - how it affects people," *Better Health Channel*, https://www.betterhealth.vic. gov.au/health/healthyliving/anger-how-it-affects-people (accessed July 9, 2024).

16 Amy McKenna, "15 Nelson Mandela Quotes," *Britannica*, https://www.britannica.c om/list/nelson-mandela-quotes (accessed August 26, 2024).

17 "pride, n.[1] meanings, etymology and more," *Oxford English Dictionary*, https://www. oed.com/dictionary/pride_n1?tl=true (accessed August 26, 2024).

18 Pope Francis, *A Gift of Joy and Hope* (2022), Worthy Publishing, p.7.

19 "Forgiveness: Your Health Depends on It," Johns Hopkins Medicine, https://www.h opkinsmedicine.org/health/wellness-and-prevention/forgiveness-your-health-de pends-on-it (accessed July 9, 2024).

A BEAUTIFUL FAITH

20 "Does the Church Teach That Anyone Who Commits Suicide Goes to Hell?," *Catholic Answers*, https://www.catholic.com/qa/i-have-been-told-that-the-catholic-church-teaches-that-anyone-who-commits-suicide-goes-to-hell (accessed July 9, 2024).

21 United States Conference of Catholic Bishops, *Ethical and religious directives for Catholic health care services*, 6th ed. (2018): 15, https://www.usccb.org/resources/et hical-religious-directives-catholic-health-service-sixth-edition-2016-06_0.pdf.

22 *Catechism of the Catholic Church*, §1700, https://www.usccb.org/sites/default/files/ flipbooks/catechism/426/ (accessed August 20, 2024).

23 *Catechism of the Catholic Church*, §2358, https://www.usccb.org/sites/default/files/ flipbooks/catechism/568/ (accessed August 26, 2024).

24 Pope Francis, *Apostolic Letter Motu Proprio Mitis Iudex Dominus Iesus by which the canons of the Code of Canon Law pertaining to cases regarding the nullity of marriage are reformed* (August 15, 2015), The Holy See, https://www.vatican.va/content/ francesco/en/motu_proprio/documents/papa-francesco-motu-proprio_201508 15_mitis-iudex-dominus-iesus.html.

25 Fulton J. Sheen, Preface to Religion (New York: Simon & Schuster, 1946), 9.

26   *Catechism of the Catholic Church*, §§2673-2676, https://www.usccb.org/sites/defau
lt/files/flipbooks/catechism/644 (accessed August 20, 2024).

27   "Scientifically Validated Miracles of Marian Apparitions," Magis Center (2021,
July 28), https://www.magiscenter.com/blog/marian-apparitions (accessed July 9,
2024).

28   "Saints," USCCB, https://www.usccb.org/offices/public-affairs/saints (accessed
July 9, 2024).

29   Kevin Symonds, *Pope Leo XIII and the Prayer to St. Michael* (San Francisco: Ignatius
Press, 2015), 45-47.

30   "Top 10 Catholic Saints Every Catholic Should Know," Catholic World Mission,
https://catholicworldmission.org/important-catholic-saints/ (accessed July 9,
2024).

31   C. Grondin, "Percentage of the Bible in the Lectionary," *Catholic Answers*, https://w
ww.catholic.com/qa/percentage-of-the-bible-in-the-lectionary (accessed July 9,
2024).

32   For more information, see the Catechism of the Catholic Church, §§1373-1377,
https://www.usccb.org/sites/default/files/flipbooks/catechism/348/ (accessed
August 26, 2024.

33   D. Frank, "Nine Proofs of the True Presence," *Catholic Exchange* (2023, May 25),
https://catholicexchange.com/nine-proofs-of-the-true-presence/ (accessed July 9,
2024).

34   ibid.

35   For further information on the original source of the term "subsists in," see the
Second Vatican Council document, *Lumen gentium no. 8*, The Holy See, https://ww
w.vatican.va/archive/hist_councils/ii_vatican_council/documents/vat-ii_const_1
9641121_lumen-gentium_en.html.

36   "subsist," *Oxford English Dictionary*, https://www.oed.com/search/dictionary/?scop
e=Entries&q=subsist (accessed August 20, 2024).

37   "Deacon-structing the One, True Church," *Salt + Light Media*, (2023, March 28), Salt
and Light Catholic Media Foundation, https://slmedia.org/blog/deacon-structing-
the-one-true-church (accessed July 9, 2024).

38   "Ask a Priest: Why Do We Say Catholicism Is the One, True Faith?," *RC Spirituality*.
https://rcspirituality.org/ask_a_priest/ask-a-priest-why-do-we-say-catholicism-i
s-the-one-true-faith/ (accessed July 9, 2024).

39   For more information, see the Catechism of the Catholic Church, §820, https://ww
w.usccb.org/sites/default/files/flipbooks/catechism/216/ (accessed 8/27/24).

40   *Joint Declaration on the Doctrine of Justification*, The Lutheran World Federation, https://lutheranworld.org/sites/default/files/Joint%20Declaration%20on%20the%20Doctrine%20of%20Justification.pdf (accessed August 21, 2024).

41   2022 Annual Report (2023, July 25), Catholic Charities USA, https://www.catholic charitiesusa.org/publications/2022-annual-report/ (accessed July 9, 2024).

42   ChatGPT, "Catholic Organizations Helping the Poor," OpenAI, accessed August 29, 2024.

43   H. F. Angel, "Revealing the Cognitive Neuroscience of Belief," *Frontiers*, https://www.frontiersin.org/journals/behavioral-neuroscience/articles/10.3389/fnbeh.2022.926742/full (accessed July 9, 2024).

LOVE ABOVE ALL

44   ibid.

45   Bishop Robert Deeley, "Admonish the Sinner," Diocese of Portland, https://portlanddiocese.org/admonish-the-sinner (accessed July 9, 2024).

46   Peter Raymond Scholtes, "They'll Know We Are Christians by Our Love," Hymnal for Young Christians (Chicago: F.E.L. Publications, 1966).

47   D. Weinstein, "Loving Yourself and Others: The Impact of Compassion on Mental Health and Wellness," VCU Health (2023, February 7), https://www.vcuhealth.org/news/loving-yourself-and-others-the-impact-of-compassion-on-mental-health-and-wellness (accessed July 9, 2024).

MAKING A POSITIVE DIFFERENCE

48   Tom Rath & Mary Reckmeyer, *How Full Is Your Bucket? For Kids*, Gallup Press (April 1, 2009).

49   For more information about the *Character Council of WNY*, visit https://characterc ouncilwny.org/.

50   Free Strengths Test, Find Your Character Traits & Personality Types, High5Test, https://high5test.com/.

51   Jeff Carver, Free Spiritual Gifts Test, https://spiritualgiftstest.com/.

MINDSET RESET

52   For more information, visit PROJECT WISDOM - Celebrating 30+ YEARS of Character Education, https://projectwisdom.com/.

53   M. Primeau, "Your powerful, changeable mindset," *Stanford Report*, (2021, September 15), https://news.stanford.edu/report/2021/09/15/mindsets-clearing-lens-life/ (accessed July 9, 2024).

54   S.J. Gillihan, "How Often Do Your Worries Actually Come True?" *Psychology Today* (2019, July 19), https://www.psychologytoday.com/intl/blog/think-act-be/201907/how-often-do-your-worries-actually-come-true (accessed July 9, 2024).

55   United States Conference of Catholic Bishops, "Communion Rite," *The Roman Missal*, Third Edition, (Washington, DC: 2011).

56   "'Nones' on the Rise in 2012," Pew Research Center (2012, October 9), https://www.pewresearch.org/religion/2012/10/09/nones-on-the-rise/ (accessed July 9, 2024).

FAITHFULLY HEALTHY

57   "Science Says: Religion Is Good For Your Health," *Forbes* (2019, March 29), https://www.forbes.com/sites/nicolefisher/2019/03/29/science-says-religion-is-good-for-your-health/?sh=2b57f30b3a12 (accessed July 9, 2024).

58   G. Lucchetti, "Spirituality, religiousness, and mental health: A review of the current scientific evidence," *NCBI*, (2021, September 16), https://www.ncbi.nlm.nih.gov/pmc/articles/PMC8462234/ (accessed July 9, 2024).

59   D. DeSteno, "Is Religion Good for Your Health?" *Wall Street Journal* (2023, June 8), https://www.wsj.com/articles/is-religion-good-for-your-health-921814a7 (accessed July 9, 2024).

60   S. Feder, "Deep faith beneficial to health," *Stanford Report* (2020, November 13), https://news.stanford.edu/stories/2020/11/deep-faith-beneficial-health (accessed July 9, 2024).

61   Kelli Harding, "Is Generosity Good for Your Health?" Columbia Doctors (2023, November 28), https://www.columbiadoctors.org/news/generosity-good-your-health (accessed July 9, 2024).

62   C. Grondin, "Will We See Our Family in Heaven?" *Catholic Answers*, https://www.catholic.com/qa/will-we-see-our-family-in-heaven (accessed July 9, 2024).

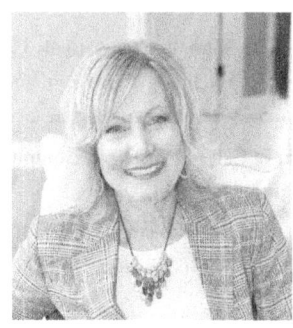

About the Author

Suzanne Bracci *has been a dedicated mental health and wellness professional since 2005, serving in various roles, including Mental Health Counselor, School Counselor, Life Coach, and Not-For-Profit President.*

In 2022, following promptings from the Holy Spirit, she stepped away from two professional positions and began integrating prayer and the Word of God into her private coaching and consulting practice. She now joyfully serves as a Christian Life & Mindset Coach, speaker, and author.

Suzanne offers complimentary resources, such as inspiring coaching devotionals and videos, as well as paid services, including her transformative 12-week H.O.P.E. Method Program, which helps women replace fear, worry, and discontentment with peace, joy, and fulfillment.

An experienced keynote speaker and workshop developer, Suzanne specializes in biblically sound natural stress and anxiety relief. She also empowers people through positive thinking strategies, effective communication, character development, healthy relationships, and personal growth.

As a school counselor, Suzanne received the 2014 Humane Educator of the Year and Teacher of the Year Awards. In 2024, she was bestowed the title of President Emerita for her leadership contributions and ten years of volunteer service to the Character Council of Western New York. Suzanne is an honored listee in the 2024 "Marquis Who's Who in America" publication for her contributions to the fields of well-being and personal growth.

She feels honored, blessed, and deeply grateful to answer God's calling to help Catholics and all people in their journeys of faith, hope, and love.

Suzanne lives in Western New York and has been married to her loving, supportive husband, Michael, for 30 years. They are proud parents of three grown children and eagerly await the arrival of their first grandchild.

For more information about Suzanne and her work, visit SuzanneBracci.com.

You can connect with me on:

🌐 https://suzannebracci.com
📘 https://www.facebook.com/SuzanneBracci.Faith.Hope.Love
📷 https://www.instagram.com/suzannebracci.faith.hope.love
🔗 https://www.linkedin.com/in/suzannebracci

Made in the USA
Monee, IL
26 September 2024

66675071R00075